Applied Meta-Analysis with R

Chapman & Hall/CRC Biostatistics Series

Chapman & Hall/CRC Biostatistics Series

Adaptive Design Methods in Clinical Trials, Second Edition
Shein-Chung Chow and Mark Chang

Adaptive Design Theory and Implementation Using SAS and R
Mark Chang

Advanced Bayesian Methods for Medical Test Accuracy
Lyle D. Broemeling

Advances in Clinical Trial Biostatistics
Nancy L. Geller

Applied Meta-Analysis with R
Ding-Geng (Din) Chen and Karl E. Peace

Basic Statistics and Pharmaceutical Statistical Applications, Second Edition
James E. De Muth

Bayesian Adaptive Methods for Clinical Trials
Scott M. Berry, Bradley P. Carlin, J. Jack Lee, and Peter Muller

Bayesian Analysis Made Simple: An Excel GUI for WinBUGS
Phil Woodward

Bayesian Methods for Measures of Agreement
Lyle D. Broemeling

Bayesian Methods in Health Economics
Gianluca Baio

Bayesian Missing Data Problems: EM, Data Augmentation and Noniterative Computation
Ming T. Tan, Guo-Liang Tian, and Kai Wang Ng

Bayesian Modeling in Bioinformatics
Dipak K. Dey, Samiran Ghosh, and Bani K. Mallick

Biostatistics: A Computing Approach
Stewart J. Anderson

Causal Analysis in Biomedicine and Epidemiology: Based on Minimal Sufficient Causation
Mikel Aickin

Clinical Trial Data Analysis using R
Ding-Geng (Din) Chen and Karl E. Peace

Clinical Trial Methodology
Karl E. Peace and Ding-Geng (Din) Chen

Computational Methods in Biomedical Research
Ravindra Khattree and Dayanand N. Naik

Computational Pharmacokinetics
Anders Källén

Confidence Intervals for Proportions and Related Measures of Effect Size
Robert G. Newcombe

Controversial Statistical Issues in Clinical Trials
Shein-Chung Chow

Data and Safety Monitoring Committees in Clinical Trials
Jay Herson

Design and Analysis of Animal Studies in Pharmaceutical Development
Shein-Chung Chow and Jen-pei Liu

Design and Analysis of Bioavailability and Bioequivalence Studies, Third Edition
Shein-Chung Chow and Jen-pei Liu

Design and Analysis of Bridging Studies
Jen-pei Liu, Shein-Chung Chow, and Chin-Fu Hsiao

Design and Analysis of Clinical Trials with Time-to-Event Endpoints
Karl E. Peace

Design and Analysis of Non-Inferiority Trials
Mark D. Rothmann, Brian L. Wiens, and Ivan S. F. Chan

Difference Equations with Public Health Applications
Lemuel A. Moyé and Asha Seth Kapadia

DNA Methylation Microarrays: Experimental Design and Statistical Analysis
Sun-Chong Wang and Arturas Petronis

DNA Microarrays and Related Genomics Techniques: Design, Analysis, and Interpretation of Experiments
David B. Allison, Grier P. Page, T. Mark Beasley, and Jode W. Edwards

Dose Finding by the Continual Reassessment Method
Ying Kuen Cheung

Elementary Bayesian Biostatistics
Lemuel A. Moyé

Frailty Models in Survival Analysis
Andreas Wienke

Generalized Linear Models: A Bayesian Perspective
Dipak K. Dey, Sujit K. Ghosh, and Bani K. Mallick

Handbook of Regression and Modeling: Applications for the Clinical and Pharmaceutical Industries
Daryl S. Paulson

Interval-Censored Time-to-Event Data: Methods and Applications
Ding-Geng (Din) Chen, Jianguo Sun, and Karl E. Peace

Joint Models for Longitudinal and Time-to-Event Data: With Applications in R
Dimitris Rizopoulos

Measures of Interobserver Agreement and Reliability, Second Edition
Mohamed M. Shoukri

Medical Biostatistics, Third Edition
A. Indrayan

Meta-Analysis in Medicine and Health Policy
Dalene Stangl and Donald A. Berry

Monte Carlo Simulation for the Pharmaceutical Industry: Concepts, Algorithms, and Case Studies
Mark Chang

Multiple Testing Problems in Pharmaceutical Statistics
Alex Dmitrienko, Ajit C. Tamhane, and Frank Bretz

Randomized Clinical Trials of Nonpharmacological Treatments
Isabelle Boutron, Philippe Ravaud, and David Moher

Randomized Phase II Cancer Clinical Trials
Sin-Ho Jung

Sample Size Calculations in Clinical Research, Second Edition
Shein-Chung Chow, Jun Shao and Hansheng Wang

Statistical Design and Analysis of Stability Studies
Shein-Chung Chow

Statistical Evaluation of Diagnostic Performance: Topics in ROC Analysis
Kelly H. Zou, Aiyi Liu, Andriy Bandos, Lucila Ohno-Machado, and Howard Rockette

Statistical Methods for Clinical Trials
Mark X. Norleans

Statistics in Drug Research: Methodologies and Recent Developments
Shein-Chung Chow and Jun Shao

Statistics in the Pharmaceutical Industry, Third Edition
Ralph Buncher and Jia-Yeong Tsay

Translational Medicine: Strategies and Statistical Methods
Dennis Cosmatos and Shein-Chung Chow

Chapman & Hall/CRC Biostatistics Series

Applied Meta-Analysis with R

Ding-Geng (Din) Chen

Karl E. Peace

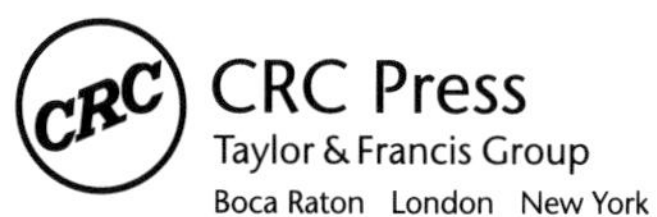

CRC Press
Taylor & Francis Group
Boca Raton London New York

CRC Press is an imprint of the
Taylor & Francis Group, an **informa** business
A CHAPMAN & HALL BOOK

CRC Press
Taylor & Francis Group
6000 Broken Sound Parkway NW, Suite 300
Boca Raton, FL 33487-2742

Printed on acid-free paper
Version Date: 20130403

International Standard Book Number-13: 978-1-4665-0599-5 (Hardback)

Visit the Taylor & Francis Web site at
http://www.taylorandfrancis.com

and the CRC Press Web site at
http://www.crcpress.com

To my parents and parents-in-law who value higher education and hard work, and to my wife, Ke, my son, John D. Chen, and my daughter, Jenny K. Chen, for their love and support.

Ding-Geng (Din) Chen

To the memory of my late mother, Elsie Mae Cloud Peace, my late wife, Jiann-Ping Hsu, and to my son, Christopher K. Peace, daughter-in-law, Ashley Hopkins Peace, and grandchildren, Camden and Henry.

Karl E. Peace

Contents

List of Figures

List of Tables

Preface

In Chapter 8 of our previous book (Chen and Peace, 2010), we briefly introduced meta-analysis using R. Since then, we have been encouraged to develop an entire book on meta-analyses using R that would include a wide variety of applications — which is the theme of this book.

In this book we provide a thorough presentation of meta-analysis with detailed step-by-step illustrations on their implementation using R. In each chapter, examples of real studies compiled from the literature and scientific publications are presented. After presenting the data and sufficient background to permit understanding of the application, various meta-analysis methods appropriate for analyzing data are identified. Then analysis code is developed using appropriate R packages and functions to meta-analyze the data. Analysis code development and results are presented in a stepwise fashion. This stepwise approach should enable readers to follow the logic and gain an understanding of the analysis methods and the R implementation so that they may use R and the steps in this book to analyze their own meta-data.

Based on their experience in biostatistical research and teaching biostatistical meta-analysis, the authors understand that there are gaps between developed statistical methods and applications of statistical methods by students and practitioners. This book is intended to fill this gap by illustrating the implementation of statistical meta-analysis methods using R applied to real data following a step-by-step presentation style.

With this style, the book is suitable as a text for a course in meta-data analysis at the graduate level (Master's or Doctorate's), particularly for students seeking degrees in statistics or biostatistics. In addition, the book should be a valuable reference for self-study and a learning tool for practitioners and biostatisticians in public health, medical research universities, governmental agencies and the pharmaceutical industry, particularly those with little or no experience in using R.

R has become widely used in statistical modeling and computing since its creation in the mid 1990s and it is now an integrated and essential software for statistical analyses. Becoming familiar with R is then imperative for the next generation of statistical data analysts. In Chapter 1, we present a basic introduction to the R system, where to get R, how to install R and how to upgrade R packages. Readers who are already familiar with R may skip this chapter and go directly to any of the remaining chapters.

In Chapter 2, we provide an overview of the research protocols for meta-analysis. In Chapter 3, we provide an overall introduction to meta-analysis for both fixed-effects and random-effects models in meta-analysis. Two real datasets are introduced along with two commonly used R packages of `meta` and `rmeta`.

In Chapters 4 and 5, we present meta-analysis for specific data types. In Chapter 4, we consider meta-analysis with binary data. We begin this chapter with two real Datasets. The first is a meta-analysis of "Statin Clinical Trials" to compare intensive statin therapy to moderate statin therapy in the reduction of cardiovascular outcomes. The second is a meta-analysis of five studies on Lamotrigine for the treatment of bipolar depression. In Chapter 5, we consider meta-analysis for continuous data. Similarly to Chapter 4, we introduce two published datasets. The first dataset uses 6 studies on the impact of intervention. The second dataset is of studies from the literature comparing tubeless to standard percutaneous nephrolithotomy.

Chapter 6 is on the development of measures to quantify heterogeneity as well as to test the significance of heterogeneity among studies in a meta-analysis. Continuing from Chapter 6 to explain heterogeneity in meta-analysis, Chapter 7 is to introduce meta-regression to explain extra heterogeneity (or the residual heterogeneity) using study-level moderators or study-level independent predictors. Three datasets are used in this chapter to illustrate the application of meta-regression with fixed-effects and random-effects meta-regressions. The first dataset contains summary information from 13 studies on the effectiveness of BCG vaccine against tuberculosis. The second dataset contains summary information from 28 studies on ischaemic heart disease (IHD) to assess the association between IHD risk reduction and reduction in serum cholesterol. Both datasets are widely used in meta-regression as examples. We recompiled a third dataset to assess whether the ability to inhibit motor responses is impaired for adolescents with attention-deficit hyperactivity disorder (ADHD). The R library `metafor` is introduced in this chapter for both meta-analysis and meta-regression.

There are extensive discussions between individual-patient data (IPD) analysis and meta-analysis (MA) in the situations where IPD are accessible. Some favor IPD and others favor MA. So in Chapter 8, we make use of actual individual-level patient data on lamotrigine (obtained from the manufacturer) to treat bipolar depression to illustrate the pros and cons of IPD and MA. Simulations are conducted in this chapter to compare IPD with MA on efficiency. All demonstrated that both models yielded very comparable results. This chapter thus serves to further promote meta-analysis using study-level summary statistics. Without much loss in relative efficiency for testing treatment effect, MA is recommended since it is usually difficult to obtain original individual-level data and is costlier and more time-consuming.

All the methods presented to Chapter 8 are based on the theory of large sample approximations. For rare events, these methods usually break down. The typical remedies are to remove the studies with zero events from the meta-analysis, or add a small value as continuity correction, say 0.5, to the rare events which usually lead to biased statistical inferences. In Chapter 9, we use the well-known Rosiglitazone meta-analysis data to illustrate the bias and then introduce a novel `confidence distributions` approach for meta-analysis where two methods are implemented for meta-analysis of rare events. We conclude the book with Chapter 10 to review other specific R packages for meta-analysis.

All R programs and datasets used in this book can be requested from Professor Ding-Geng (Din) Chen at DrDG.Chen@gmail.com. Readers can refer to Section 1.3 to load the specific data from the Excel databook into R. Also readers may use and modify the R programs for their own applications. To facilitate the understanding of implementation in R, we annotated all the R programs with comments and explanations starting with `#` (i.e. the R command for "comment") so that the readers can understand exactly the meaning of the corresponding R programs. Note that some of the R outputs are reformatted and modified to fit the pages and figures in finalizing the entire LaTeX document.

We would like to express our gratitude to many individuals. First, thanks to David Grubbs from Taylor & Francis for his interest in the book and to Shashi Kumar for assistance in LaTeX. Also thanks to Dr. Gary Evoniuk (GlaxoSmithKline, NC), Ms. Suzanne Edwards (GlaxoSmithKline, NC) and Dr. Dungang Liu (Yale University, CT) for their suggestions and comments to Chapter 8, and to Professor Minge Xie (Rutgers University, NJ), Drs. Dungang Liu (Yale University, CT) and Guang Yang (Rutgers University, NJ) for their suggestions and comments to Chapter 9 as well as their wonderful job to produce the R package `gmeta`. Of course we very much thank GlaxoSmithKline for providing and permitting use of the actual data in Chapter 9.

Special thanks are due to Professors Robert Gentleman and Ross Ihaka who created the R language with visionary open source, as well as to the developers and contributing authors in the R community for their endless efforts and contributed packages.

Finally, thanks go to Xinyan (Abby) Yan, our graduate assistant, for her dedicated and valuable assistance in compiling datasets, and to Dr. Nicole Trabold (University of Rochester, NY) for her careful reading of the book.

We welcome any comments and suggestions on typos, errors and future improvements about this book. Please contact Professor Ding-Geng (Din) Chen at email: DrDG.Chen@gmail.com.

Rochester, NY, Ding-Geng (Din) Chen
Statesboro, GA, Karl E. Peace

December 12, 2012

Chapter 1

Introduction to R

In this chapter, we begin with a basic introduction to the R system: where to get R, how to install R and upgrade R packages. We also show how easy it is to use R for data management as well as to simulate and analyze data from multi-center studies with a brief introduction to meta-analysis. We conclude the chapter with a brief summary and some recommendations for further reading and references.

The main goal for this chapter is to introduce R to readers. For readers who already know and have familiarity with R, you can skip this chapter and go directly to any of the remaining chapters.

1.1 What is R?

R was initially created by Ihaka and Gentleman (1996) from University of Auckland, New Zealand. Since its creation in the middle of the 1990s, R has quickly become a popular programming language and an environment for statistical computing. The continuing development of R is carried out by a core team from different institutions around the world.

To obtain an introduction to R, go to the official home page of the R project at

http://www.R-project.org

and click "What is R?":

"R is a language and environment for statistical computing

and graphics. It is a GNU project which is similar to the S language and environment which was developed at Bell Laboratories (formerly AT&T, now Lucent Technologies) by John Chambers and colleagues. R can be considered as a different implementation of S. There are some important differences, but much code written for S runs unaltered under R.

R provides a wide variety of statistical (linear and nonlinear modelling, classical statistical tests, time-series analysis, classification, clustering, ...) and graphical techniques, and is highly extensible. The S language is often the vehicle of choice for research in statistical methodology, and R provides an Open Source route to participation in that activity.

One of R's strengths is the ease with which well-designed publication-quality plots can be produced, including mathematical symbols and formulae where needed. Great care has been taken over the defaults for the minor design choices in graphics, but the user retains full control.

R is available as Free Software under the terms of the Free Software Foundation's GNU General Public License in source code form. It compiles and runs on a wide variety of UNIX platforms and similar systems (including FreeBSD and Linux), Windows and MacOS."

To some users, "free" software may be a "negative" word for software that is difficult to use, has lower quality or utilizes procedures that have not been validated or verified, etc. However, to other users, "free" software means software from an open source that not only allows use of the software but also permits modifications to handle a variety of applications. This latter description is the fundamental principle for R system.

We now proceed to the steps for installing and using R.

1.2 Steps for Installing R and Updating R Packages

In general, the R system consists of two parts. One is the so-called R *base system* for the core R language and associated fundamental libraries. The other consists of user contributed *packages* that are more specialized applications. Both the *base system* and the *packages* may be obtained from the Comprehensive R Archive Network (CRAN) from the weblink:

`http://CRAN.r-project.org`

Installation of the R system is described in the following sections.

1.2.1 First Step: Install R *Base System*

The *base system* can be downloaded from

`http://CRAN.r-project.org`

for different platforms of "Linux", "MacOS" and "Windows". In this book, we illustrate the use of R for "Windows". "Windows" users can download the latest version of R using the link:

`http://CRAN.r-project.org/bin/windows/base/release.htm`

(At the writing of this book, version *R 2.5.1* is available.). To download and install R to your computer simply follow the instructions from the installer to install R to the "Program Files" subdirectory in your C. You are ready to use R for statistical computing and data analysis.

Note to LaTeX and *R/Sweave* users: LaTeX will complain about the extra space in the path as in "Program Files". Therefore if you want to use R along with LaTeX, you need to make a subdirectory *without* space in the path to install R.

You should now have an icon with shortcut to R. Simply click the icon to start R. You should see some introductory information about R and a command prompt '>':

```
>
```

To illustrate R computation, suppose we wish to calculate the sum of 1 and 2012. The first line of R computation is:

```
> x = 1+2012
```

The computed value may be printed using:

```
> print(x)
```

```
[1] 2013
```

You should get "2013".

1.2.2 Second Step: Installing and Updating R Packages

The R *base system* contains a variety of standard statistical functions, descriptive and inferential statistical analysis methods, and graphics which are appropriate for many statistical computing and data analysis requirements.

However, the *packages* are more specialized applications that are contributed by advanced R users who are expert in their field. From our view, *packages* in R is the most important component in R development and upgrading. At the time of writing this book, there are more than 5000 packages in the R system spanning almost all fields of statistical computing and methodology which can be downloaded from `http://cran.r-project.org/web/packages/`. For reassurance, we can say that you can find anything you need in R.

You may install any *packages* from the R prompt by clicking `install.packages` from the R menu *Packages* .

For example, for researchers and practitioners who are interested in meta-analysis, there are several R packages for this purpose, such as the *meta*, *rmeta*, and *metafor* which can be installed from this pull-down manual. All the functionality of this package is then available by loading it to R as:

```
> # Load the `meta' package
> library(meta)
> # Load `rmeta' package
> library(rmeta)
> # Load `metafor' package
> library(metafor)
```

For first-time users for this package, information about its use may be obtained by invoking the 'help' manual, such as:

```
> library(help=metafor)
```

A help page is then available which explains all the functionality of this package. For readers who desire a comprehensive list of available packages, go to

`http://CRAN.R-project.org/src/contrib/PACKAGES.html`

1.2.3 Steps to Get Help and Documentation

A striking feature of R is the easy access of its "Help and Documentation" which may distinguish it from other software systems. There are several ways to access "Help and Documentation".

A general help for R can be obtained by typing `help.start` where you can find help on

1. `Manuals` on
   - An Introduction to R
   - The R Language Definition
   - Writing R Extensions
   - R Installation and Administration
   - R Data Import/Export
   - R Internals
2. `Reference`
   - Packages
   - Search Engine & Keywords
3. `Miscellaneous Material`
   - About R
   - Authors
   - Resources

- License
- Frequently Asked Questions
- Thanks
- NEWS
- User Manuals
- Technical papers

4. `Material specific to the Windows port`

- CHANGES
- Windows FAQ

A general reference may be obtained from *RGui* in R. When R is started, click "Help" to access R help items on "FAQ on R", "FAQ on R on Windows", "Manuals (in PDF)", etc. We recommend that readers print the online PDF manual "Introduction to R" for future reference.

Additional "Help and Documentation" may be obtained from the R Homepage. Documentations and online discussion about R are available from the R homepage `http://www.r-project.org/`. The online "Documentation" section consists of almost all the manuals, FAQs, R Journal, books and other related information. We recommend readers spend some time in reviewing the online documents to gain familiarity with R.

The most convenient way to access 'Help' is from the R command prompt. You can always obtain specific help information from the R command prompt by using "help()". For example, if you want help on "Calculate Effect Size and Outcome Measures" in the library *metafor*, type:

```
> help(escalc)
```

This will load an information page on "Calculate Effect Size and Outcome Measures" containing relevant information. This includes the description of the function, detailed usage for the function and some examples on how to use this function.

1.3 Database Management and Data Manipulations

1.3.1 RMySQL to Microsoft Excel

There are several packages in R for database management and data manipulations. One of the most popular databases used with R is MySQL which is freely available at http://mysql.com for a variety of platforms and is relatively easy to configure and operate. Corresponding to MySQL, there is a R package RMYSQL which is maintained by Jeffrey Horner and available at http://cran.r-project.org/web/packages/RMySQL/. For readers who are familiar with MySQL and relational databases, we highly recommend this R package to create tables and store data into MySQL.

In writing this book, we make use of the familiar Microsoft Excel spreadsheet structures and have created Excel datasheets for each dataset used in each chapter. So we will introduce R functionalities to read Excel data.

There are several ways to access Excel databook. In writing Chen and Peace (2010) we used R package RODBC (i.e. R for Open DataBase Connectivity) to read data from Excel databook to R with the odbcConnectExcel and odbcConnectExcel2007 since at that time, our computer system is 32-bit. This package is available at http://cran.r-project.org/web/packages/RODBC/.

Since 64-bit computers have more or less replaced those 32-bit computers, in this book we introduce gdata, another more general R package to read the data from Excel databook. This package is available at http://cran.r-project.org/web/packages/gdata/. As an alternative to the functions in the RODBC package, the function of read.xls in gdata can be used to read an Excel datasheet into R. Since this function is linked to a module from perl language (http://perl.org), you are required to install perl first into your computer. This can be easily done from http://perl.org; for example we install perl at path "c:/perl64". With installed perl, read.xls translates the Excel spreadsheet into a comma-separated values (CSV) file, and then calls another R function read.csv to read the .csv file.

For example, to read the data in Statin Clinical Trials to be used in Section 4.1.1, the R code chunk is as follows:

```
> # Load the library
> require(gdata)
> # Link to the Excel Databook at your file path
> datfile = "Your Data Path/dat4Meta.xls"
> # Call "read.xls" to read the specific Excel data sheet
> dat   = read.xls(datfile, sheet="Data_Statin2006",
                perl="c:/perl64/bin/perl.exe")
> # Print the data
> print(dat)
```

```
     Study nhigh evhigh nstd evstd  ntot evtot
1 Prove It  2099    147 2063   172  4162   319
2   A-to-Z  2265    205 2232   235  4497   440
3      TNT  4995    334 5006   418 10001   752
4    IDEAL  4439    411 4449   463  8888   874
```

We use this structure in this book to read the data from the Excel databook we created in writing this book. We recommend readers gain familiarity with this format. Note that you will need to specify your file path at your computer where you store the Excel databook, i.e. change "Your Data Path" to where you store "dat4Meta.xls".

1.3.2 Other Methods to Read Data into R

If you have Microsoft Excel in your computer, the easiest way to access the data is to export the data into a tab-delimited or comma-separated form, and use `read.table` or `read.csv` to import the data into R.

The `read.table` function is a generic and flexible function used to read data into R in the form of a dataframe. To get familiar with its full functionality, use 'help' as follows:

```
> help(read.table)
```

You will see the description and detailed usage. Examples are given on how to use this function. Some of the functionalities are reiterated here for easy reference:

- `header=TRUE`: If the first line in the data is the variable names, the `header=TRUE` argument is used in `read.table` to use these names to identify the columns of the output dataframe. Otherwise `read.table` would just name the variables using a `V` followed by the column number. In this case, we can use `col.names=` argument in `read.table` to specify a name vector for the dataframe.

- `row.names=`: The `row.names` argument is used to name the rows in the dataframe from `read.table`. Without `row.names` or with `row.names=NULL`, the rows in the dataframe will be listed as the observations numbers.

- `Missing Values`: As its default, `read.table` automatically treats the symbol `NA` to represent a missing value for any data type. For numeric data, `NaN`, `Inf` and `-Inf` will be treated as missing. If other structure is used for missing values, the `na.strings` argument should be used to refer to that structure to represent missing values.

- `skip=`: The `skip=` argument is used to control the number of lines to skip at the beginning of the file to be read, which is useful in situations where the data have imbedded explanation at the beginning. For a very large datafile, we can specify `nrows=` argument to limit the maximum number of rows to read and increase the speed of data processing.

As wrappers for `read.table`, there are three functions of `read.csv`, `read.csv2` and `read.delim` used specifically for comma-, semicolon-, or tab-delimited data, respectively.

1.3.3 R Package `foreign`

For other data formats, the R core team created a package called Rcmdforeign, to read and write data from other statistical packages, such as: Minitab, S, SAS, SPSS, Stata, Systat and dBase. This package is available at `http://cran.r-project.org/web/packages/foreign/` with a detailed manual at `http://cran.r-project.org/web/packages/foreign/foreign.pdf` to describe its functionalities.

1.4 A Simple Simulation on Multi-Center Studies

To demonstrate basic application of R and its functionality, we simulate a simple multi-center study to compare a new antihypertensive drug (denoted by `Drug`) to a conventional control drug (denoted by `CTRL`) on reducing diastolic blood pressure in hypertensive adult men.

Let's assume an appropriate power analysis indicated that the sample size required to detect a specified treatment difference is $n = 1,000$. Since it is difficult to recruit 1,000 participants at one location during the specified time frame, the research team decided to conduct a multi-center study to recruit these participants from five centers, which led to a five-center study. For these n participants, we record their age and measure baseline diastolic blood pressure just before randomization since *age* is an important risk factor linked to blood pressure.

The new and the control drugs are administered and blood pressure is measured and recorded periodically thereafter, including at the end of the study. Then the change in blood pressure between the endpoint and baseline may be calculated and used to evaluate the antihypertensive efficacy of the new drug.

We illustrate the simulation of the data, data manipulation and analysis with appropriate statistical graphics. Since this is the very first introduction to R, we intentionally use the basic R command so that readers can follow the logic without difficulty.

1.4.1 Data Simulation

1.4.1.1 R Functions

R has a wide range of functions to handle probability distributions and data simulation. For example, for the commonly used normal distribution, its *Density, cumulative distribution function, quantile function* and *random generation* with mean equal to *mean* and standard deviation equal to *sd* can be generated using the following R functions:

```
dnorm(x, mean = 0, sd = 1, log = FALSE)
```

```
pnorm(q, mean = 0, sd = 1, lower.tail = TRUE, log.p = FALSE)
qnorm(p, mean = 0, sd = 1, lower.tail = TRUE, log.p = FALSE)
rnorm(n, mean = 0, sd = 1)
```

where

x, q	*is*	vector of quantiles
p	*is*	vector of probabilities
n	*is*	number of observations
mean	*is*	vector of means
sd	*is*	vector of standard deviations.

The above specification can be found using the *Help* function as follows:

```
> help(rnorm)
```

There are similar sets of *d*, *p*, *q*, *r* functions for *Poisson*, *binomial*, *t*, *F*, *hypergeometric*, χ^2, *Beta*, etc. Also there is a *sample* function for sampling from a vector *replicate* for repeating computations.

1.4.1.2 Data Generation and Manipulation

With this introduction, we can now simulate data center-by-center. For example in center 1, let's assume that the baseline diastolic blood pressures for these 200 (n=100 for each treatment) recruited participants are normally distributed with mean (mu) = 100 (mmHg) and standard deviation sd = 20 (mmHg). The *age* for these 200 middle-age men is assumed to be normally distributed with mean age $age.mu$ = 50 (year old) and standard deviation $age.sd$ = 10 (year). In addition, we assume the new drug will decrease diastolic blood pressure by $mu.d$ = 20(mmHg).

These input values at center 1 for this simulation can be specified in R as follows:

```
> # Number of participants each arm
> n      = 100
> # Mean blood pressure at baseline
> mu     = 100
> # Standard deviations for blood pressure
```

```
> sd      = 20
> # Mean changes for blood pressure
> mu.d    = 10
> # Mean age for participants
> age.mu = 50
> # sd of age for participants
> age.sd = 10
```

We first simulate data for the n *CTRL* participants with *age*, baseline blood pressure (denoted by *bp.base*), endpoint blood pressure (denoted by *bp.end*) and change in blood pressure from baseline to endpoint (denoted by *bp.diff=bp.end-bp.base*) with the following R code chunk:

```
> # Fix the seed for random number generation
> set.seed(123)
> # Use "rnorm" to generate random normal
> age          = rnorm(n, age.mu, age.sd)
> bp.base      = rnorm(n,mu,sd)
> bp.end       = rnorm(n,mu,sd)
> # Take the difference between endpoint and baseline
> bp.diff      = bp.end-bp.base
> # put the data together using "cbind" to column-bind
> dat4CTRL     = round(cbind(age,bp.base,bp.end,bp.diff))
```

Note that the simulation seed is set at 123 so that simulation can be reproduced, which is done by `set.seed(123)`. Otherwise, results can be different from each simulation.

We can manipulate the data using column bind (R command `cbind`) to combine all the simulated data together and round the data into the nearest whole number (R command `round`) to produce a dataset and give the data matrix a name: *dat4CTRL*. The first few observations may be viewed using the following R code:

```
> head(dat4CTRL)

     age bp.base bp.end bp.diff
[1,]  44      86    144      58
```

```
[2,]  48    105   126    21
[3,]  66     95    95     0
[4,]  51     93   111    18
[5,]  51     81    92    11
[6,]  67     99    90    -9
```

Similarly, we can simulate data for the new drug *Drug*. We use the same variable names here, but give a different name to the final dataset: *dat4drug*. Note that the *mean* for the *bp.end* is now *mu-mu.d* to simulate the decrease in mean value:

```
> # Simulate `age'
> age      = rnorm(n, age.mu, age.sd)
> # Simulate `baseline' blood pressure
> bp.base  = rnorm(n,mu,sd)
> # Simulate `endpoint' blood pressure
> bp.end   = rnorm(n,mu-mu.d,sd)
> # The changes in blood pressure
> bp.diff  = bp.end-bp.base
> # Make the data matrix
> dat4drug = round(cbind(age,bp.base,bp.end,bp.diff))
```

We do not print the observations at this time. To further manipulate the data, we stack the two datasets from *CTRL* and *Drug* using R command `rbind` to produce a dataframe using R command `data.frame`. We also create a column *TRT* with two factors of *CTRL* and *Drug* to indicate there are two treatments in this dataset and another column *Center* to represent the data is from which center. Finally we name this data as *dat1*:

```
> # Make a dataframe to hold all data
> dat1     = data.frame(rbind(dat4CTRL,dat4drug))
> # Make "TRT" as a factor for treatment.
> dat1$TRT    = as.factor(rep(c("CTRL", "Drug"), each=n))
> # Make a "Center" to represent the center number
> dat1$Center = 1
```

With these manipulations, the dataframe *dat1* should have 200 observations with 100 from *CTRL* and 100 from *Drug*. Also this dataframe should have 6 *age, bp.base, bp.end, bp.diff, TRT, Center* as columns. We can check it using the following R code chunk:

```
> # check the data dimension
> dim(dat1)
```

```
[1] 200   6
```

```
> # print the first 6 obervations to see the variable names
> head(dat1)
```

```
  age bp.base bp.end bp.diff  TRT Center
1  44      86    144      58 CTRL      1
2  48     105    126      21 CTRL      1
3  66      95     95       0 CTRL      1
4  51      93    111      18 CTRL      1
5  51      81     92      11 CTRL      1
6  67      99     90      -9 CTRL      1
```

We can then write this process of data generation into a function so that we can call this function to simulate data for other centers. We name this function as *data.generator* as follows:

```
> data.generator = function(n,age.mu,age.sd,mu,mu.d,sd, center){
 # Data from CTRL
 age      = rnorm(n, age.mu, age.sd)
 bp.base  = rnorm(n,mu,sd)
 bp.end   = rnorm(n,mu,sd)
 bp.diff  = bp.end-bp.base
 dat4CTRL = round(cbind(age,bp.base,bp.end,bp.diff))
 # Data from Drug
 age      = rnorm(n, age.mu, age.sd)
 bp.base  = rnorm(n,mu,sd)
 bp.end   = rnorm(n,mu-mu.d,sd)
 bp.diff  = bp.end-bp.base
 dat4drug = round(cbind(age,bp.base,bp.end,bp.diff))
 # Put both data matrice\tilde{}s together
 dat      = data.frame(rbind(dat4CTRL,dat4drug))
```

```
# Make "TRT" as a factor for treatment.
dat$TRT   = as.factor(rep(c("CTRL", "Drug"), each=n))
# Make a "Center" to represent the center number
dat$Center   = center
# Return the simulated data
dat
} # end of function
```

With this new function of `data.generator`, we can re-generate the data from center 1 as follows:

```
> d1 = data.generator(n,age.mu,age.sd,mu,mu.d,sd, 1)
```

To generate data from other centers, we suppose mean and standard deviation for baseline blood pressure and age are similar for all centers, but the new drug has different effectiveness for each center with `mu.d2 = 13` for center 2, `mu.d3 = 15` for center 3, `mu.d4 = 8` for center 4 and `mu.d5 = 10` for center 5, respectively. Then we can generate data from each center as follows:

```
> # Data from Center 2
> mu.d2 = 13
> d2     = data.generator(n,age.mu,age.sd,mu,mu.d2,sd,2)
> # Data from Center 3
> mu.d3 = 15
> d3     = data.generator(n,age.mu,age.sd,mu,mu.d3,sd,3)
> # Data from Center 4
> mu.d4 = 8
> d4     = data.generator(n,age.mu,age.sd,mu,mu.d4,sd,4)
> # Data from Center 5
> mu.d5 = 10
> d5     = data.generator(n,age.mu,age.sd,mu,mu.d5,sd,5)
```

Putting these data from 5 centers together, we create one dataset for this study which is named as `dat` as follows:

```
> dat          = data.frame(rbind(d1,d2,d3,d4,d5))
> # Change `Center' from numeric to factor
> dat$Center = as.factor(dat$Center)
```

This data should have 1000 observations from 5 centers, each having 100 from *CTRL* and 100 from *Drug*. Also this dataframe should have 6 *age, bp.base, bp.end, bp.diff, TRT, Center* as columns.

1.4.1.3 Basic R Graphics

R is well-known for its graphics capabilities. We can display the distributions for the data just generated to view whether they appear to be normally distributed using the R command `boxplot` for the first center as follows:

```
> # call boxplot
> boxplot(dat4CTRL, las=1, main="Control Drug")
```

This will generate Figure 1.1 from which one can see that the data appear to be normally distributed except for one outlier from the baseline data.

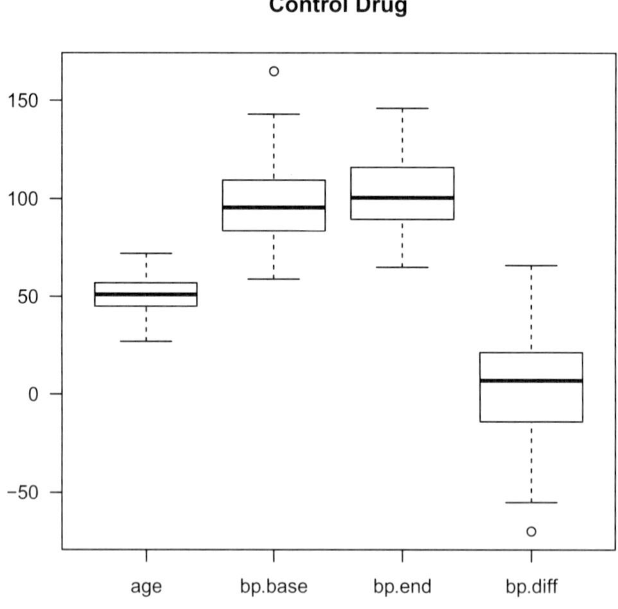

FIGURE 1.1: Distributions for Data Generated for "Control Drug"

Similarly we can produce the distribution for *Drug* using the following R code chunk:

```
> boxplot(dat4drug, las=1, main="New Drug")
```

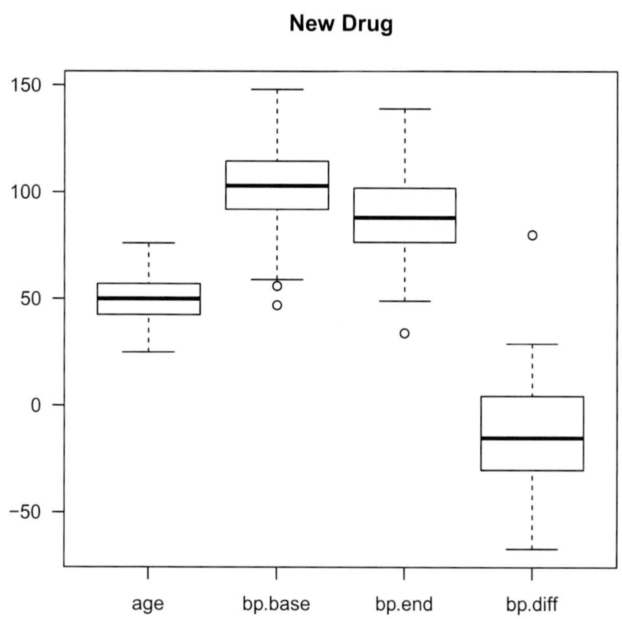

FIGURE 1.2: Distributions for Data Generated for "New Drug"

This will produce Figure 1.2 to show that the data are in fact normally distributed. The boxplot for endpoint is 10 mmHG lower than the baseline blood pressure.

Before performing any statistical analysis, we recommend exploring the data using appropriate plots to assess whether distributional or other relevant assumptions required for the validity of the analysis methods hold for the data. There is another suite of advanced R graphics to use for this purpose, i.e. the package *lattice* with implementation of Trellis Graphics.

This package is maintained by Deepayan Sarkar (Sarkar (2008)) and can be downloaded from

http://r-forge.r-project.org/projects/lattice/

or simply from RGUI. We first load the package into R by `library(lattice)` and display the relationship between the blood pressure difference as a function of *age* for each treatment to assess whether there exists a statistically significant relationship in addition to a treatment difference. This can be done with the following R code chunk:

```
> #load the lattice library
> library(lattice)
> # call xyplot function and print it
> print(xyplot(bp.diff~age|Center*TRT, data=dat,xlab="Age",
 strip=strip.custom(bg="white"),
 ylab="Blood Pressure Difference",lwd=3,cex=1.3,pch=20,
 type=c("p", "r")))
```

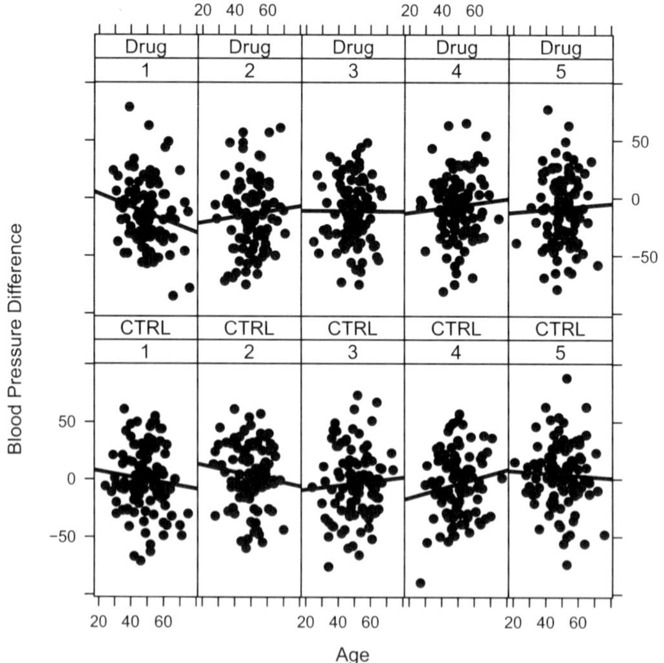

FIGURE 1.3: Data with Regression Line for Each Treatment and Center

This produces Figure 1.3. From Figure 1.3, we conclude that the relationship between the blood pressure decrease and age is not significant, but that the new drug did reduce blood pressure.

To illustrate the treatment effect by center, we can make use of the `bwplot` in this `lattice` library to produce Figure 1.4.

```
> # Call bwplot
> print(bwplot(bp.diff~TRT|Center, data=dat,xlab="TRT",
 strip=strip.custom(bg="white"),
 ylab="Blood Pressure Difference",lwd=3,cex=1.3,pch=20,
 type=c("p", "r")))
```

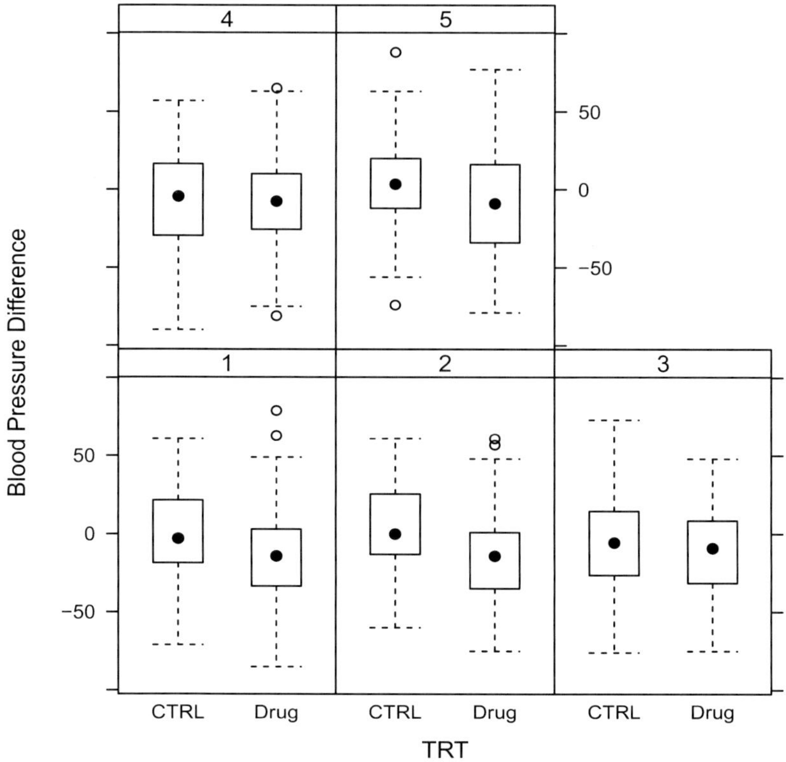

FIGURE 1.4: Treatment Effect by Center

Another way to illustrate the treatment effect is to group the treatment by center which can be produced in Figure 1.5 with the following R code chunk. We can see there are some variations within centers which is exactly what we simulated with different mu.d.

```
> # Call bwplot
> print(bwplot(bp.diff~Center|TRT, data=dat,xlab="Center",
 strip=strip.custom(bg="white"),
 ylab="Blood Pressure Difference",lwd=3,cex=1.3,pch=20,
 type=c("p", "r")))
```

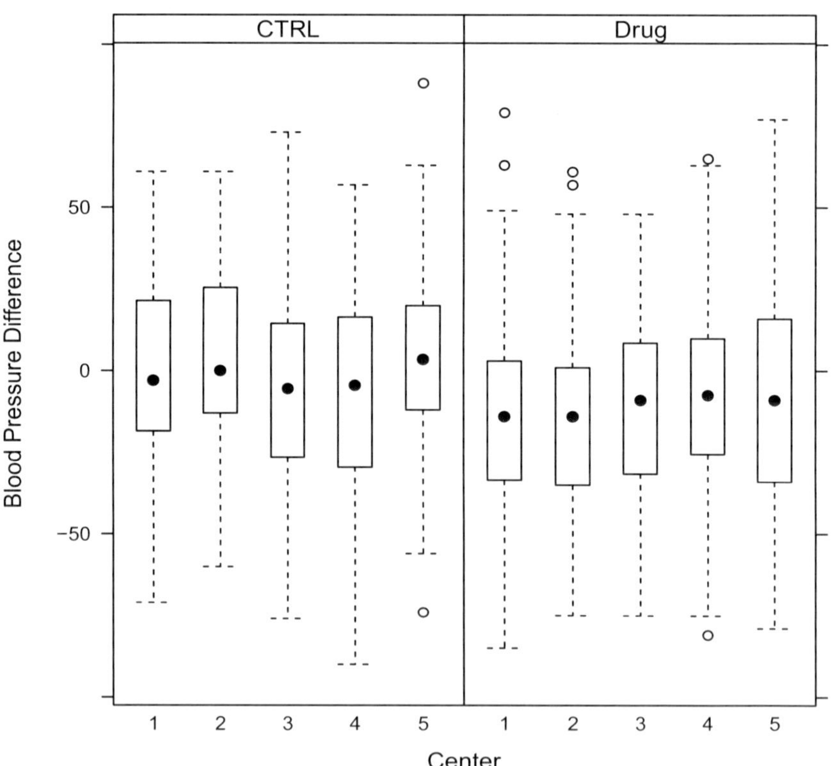

FIGURE 1.5: Treatment Effect Grouped by Center

1.4.2 Data Analysis

With these preliminary graphical illustrations, we now comfortably proceed to data analysis. We will compare the treatment effect with results using data from each individual center as well as the results from pooled data from five centers. We will then briefly introduce the concept of meta-analysis with this simulated data.

1.4.2.1 Data Analysis from Each Center

Alternatively we may perform a pooled analysis across centers by starting with the individual center effects where we would expect less statistically significant results. That is, we subset the data from each center to perform an analysis of variance using the following R code chunk:

```
> # Model for Center 1
> m.c1 = aov(bp.diff~TRT, data=dat[dat$Center==1,])
> # Print the summary
> summary(m.c1)
```

```
             Df Sum Sq Mean Sq F value Pr(>F)
TRT           1   7963    7963    9.56 0.0023 **
Residuals   198 164958     833
---
Signif. codes:  0 `***' 0.001 `**' 0.01 `*' 0.05 `.' 0.1 ` ' 1
```

```
> # Model for Center 2
> m.c2 = aov(bp.diff~TRT, data=dat[dat$Center==2,])
> # Print the summary
> summary(m.c2)
```

```
             Df Sum Sq Mean Sq F value  Pr(>F)
TRT           1  14775   14775    17.7 3.9e-05 ***
Residuals   198 165407     835
---
Signif. codes:  0 `***' 0.001 `**' 0.01 `*' 0.05 `.' 0.1 ` ' 1
```

```
> # Model for Center 3
> m.c3 = aov(bp.diff~TRT, data=dat[dat$Center==3,])
```

```
> # Print the summary
> summary(m.c3)

             Df Sum Sq Mean Sq F value Pr(>F)
TRT           1   2880    2880    3.48  0.064 .
Residuals   198 164018     828
---
Signif. codes:  0 `***' 0.001 `**' 0.01 `*' 0.05 `.' 0.1 ` ' 1

> # Model for Center 4
> m.c4 = aov(bp.diff~TRT, data=dat[dat$Center==4,])
> # Print the summary
> summary(m.c4)

             Df Sum Sq Mean Sq F value Pr(>F)
TRT           1    341     341    0.42   0.52
Residuals   198 159168     804

> # Model for Center 5
> m.c5 = aov(bp.diff~TRT, data=dat[dat$Center==5,])
> # Print the summary
> summary(m.c5)

             Df Sum Sq Mean Sq F value Pr(>F)
TRT           1   7951    7951    9.14 0.0028 **
Residuals   198 172241     870
---
Signif. codes:  0 `***' 0.001 `**' 0.01 `*' 0.05 `.' 0.1 ` ' 1
```

From these fittings, as an aside we notice that the treatment effect is statistically significant (at p-value <0.05) for centers 1, 2 and 5, but not for centers 3 and 4.

1.4.2.2 Data Analysis with Pooled Data from five-Centers

To pool all the data from the 5 centers, we start to fit a full model with 3-way interactions among treatment, Center and covariate as follows:

$$\begin{aligned} y &= \beta_0 + \beta_1 TRT + \beta_2 Center + \beta_3 age \\ &+ \beta_4 TRT \times Center + \beta_5 TRT \times age + \beta_6 Center \times age \\ &+ \beta_7 TRT \times Center \times age + \epsilon \end{aligned} \tag{1.1}$$

where y denotes the change in blood pressure and β's are the parameters. ϵ is the error term which is assumed to be independently identically distributed ($i.i.d.$) with normal distribution with standard deviation σ.

The fitting of this linear model (1.1) is accomplished in one line of R code using aov as:

```
> # Call 'aov' to fit the 3-way model
> lm1 = aov(bp.diff~TRT*Center*age, data=dat)
> summary(lm1)

               Df Sum Sq Mean Sq F value  Pr(>F)
TRT             1  27689   27689   33.17 1.1e-08 ***
Center          4   2978     745    0.89    0.47
age             1     71      71    0.08    0.77
TRT:Center      4   6194    1548    1.85    0.12
TRT:age         1      9       9    0.01    0.92
Center:age      4   5391    1348    1.61    0.17
TRT:Center:age  4   2261     565    0.68    0.61
Residuals     980 818088     835
---
Signif. codes:  0 `***' 0.001 `**' 0.01 `*' 0.05 `.' 0.1 ` ' 1
```

The summary prints a summary of the model fitting including the analysis of variance (ANOVA) table, and we can see that there are no statistically significant 3-way and 2-way interactions. So we drop the age covariate and refit a reduced model with Center as block to pool the data from 5 centers. This model can be expressed as

$$y = \beta_0 + \beta_1 TRT + \beta_2 Center + \epsilon \tag{1.2}$$

And the R implementation can be done as follows:

```
> # Call 'aov' to fit the reduced model
> lm2 = aov(bp.diff~TRT+Center, data=dat)
> summary(lm2)
```

```
            Df Sum Sq Mean Sq F value  Pr(>F)
TRT          1  27689   27689   33.08 1.2e-08 ***
Center       4   2978     745    0.89    0.47
Residuals  994 832014     837
---
Signif. codes:  0 `***' 0.001 `**' 0.01 `*' 0.05 `.' 0.1 ` ' 1
```

It can be seen from the output that there is a statistically significant treatment effect with data pooled from 5 centers which confirmed with the illustration from Figure 1.5 that the new drug statistically significantly reduced blood pressure.

1.4.2.3 A Brief Introduction to Meta-Analysis

As an alternative to the pooled multi-center analysis in the previous section, we will briefly introduce the concept of meta-analysis. We will make use of the R library `metafor` indexR Packages! metafor which will be illustrated in later chapters.

In order to carry out a meta-analysis, we first need to `aggregate` the individual data by study for their sample size, means and standard deviations which can be done with following R code chunk:

```
> # Get the study sample size
> ndat = aggregate(dat$bp.diff,
      list(Center=dat$Center,TRT = dat$TRT), length)
> # Print the study specific sample size
> ndat
```

```
   Center  TRT   x
1       1 CTRL 100
2       2 CTRL 100
3       3 CTRL 100
```

```
4         4 CTRL 100
5         5 CTRL 100
6         1 Drug 100
7         2 Drug 100
8         3 Drug 100
9         4 Drug 100
10        5 Drug 100

> # Calcuate the means by study
> mdat = aggregate(dat$bp.diff,
     list(Center=dat$Center,TRT = dat$TRT), mean)
> # Print the means
> mdat

   Center  TRT      x
1       1 CTRL  -0.24
2       2 CTRL   3.05
3       3 CTRL  -3.84
4       4 CTRL  -4.43
5       5 CTRL   3.84
6       1 Drug -12.86
7       2 Drug -14.14
8       3 Drug -11.43
9       4 Drug  -7.04
10      5 Drug  -8.77

> # Calculate the standard deviations
> sddat = aggregate(dat$bp.diff,
     list(Center=dat$Center,TRT = dat$TRT), sd)
> # Print the SDs
> sddat

   Center  TRT    x
1       1 CTRL 29.2
2       2 CTRL 27.4
3       3 CTRL 30.0
4       4 CTRL 28.3
```

```
5          5 CTRL 28.3
6          1 Drug 28.5
7          2 Drug 30.3
8          3 Drug 27.5
9          4 Drug 28.4
10         5 Drug 30.6
```

To carry out the meta-analysis, we load the `metafor` library and calculate the effect-size using mean-difference as follows:

```
> # Call the library
> library(metafor)
> # Calculate the ESs
> esdat = escalc(measure="MD",
        n1i= ndat$x[ndat$TRT=="Drug"],
    n2i= ndat$x[ndat$TRT=="CTRL"],
        m1i= mdat$x[mdat$TRT=="Drug"],
    m2i= mdat$x[mdat$TRT=="CTRL"],
        sd1i= sddat$x[sddat$TRT=="Drug"],
    sd2i= sddat$x[sddat$TRT=="CTRL"], append=T)
> rownames(esdat) = ndat$Study[ndat$TRT=="TRT"]
> # Print the ES dataframe
> esdat
```

```
      yi   vi
1 -12.62 16.7
2 -17.19 16.7
3  -7.59 16.6
4  -2.61 16.1
5 -12.61 17.4
```

With this calculated ES as mean-difference, we can then calculate the study-specific p-values as follows:

```
> # Calculate the z-values for each study
> z = esdat$yi/sqrt(esdat$vi)
> # Calculate the p-values for each study
```

```
> pval.studywise = 2*(1-pnorm(abs(z)))
> # Print the p-values
> pval.studywise

[1] 0.00199 0.0000261 0.0622 0.515 0.00250
```

This result is similar to the results from the ANOVAs in Section 1.4.2.1 which concludes that the treatment effect is statistically significant (at p-value <0.05) for centers 1, 2 and 5, but not for centers 3 and 4.

For meta-analysis, we use a random-effects meta-model with DerSimonian-Laird estimator which will be explained in the later chapter using following R code chunk:

```
> # Random-effects meta-analysis with DL
> meta.MD.DL = rma(yi,vi,measure="MD",method="DL", data=esdat)
> # Print the result
> meta.MD.DL

Random-Effects Model (k = 5; tau^2 estimator: DL)

tau^2 (estimate of total amount of heterogeneity): 14.9509
tau (sqrt of the estimate of total heterogeneity): 3.8666
I^2 (% of total variability due to heterogeneity): 47.27%
H^2 (total variability / sampling variability):    1.90

Test for Heterogeneity:
Q(df = 4) = 7.5865, p-val = 0.1080

Model Results:

estimate       se      zval      pval     ci.lb     ci.ub

-10.4810   2.5151   -4.1673   <.0001  -15.4104   -5.5515     ***
---
Signif. codes:  0 `***' 0.001 `**' 0.01 `*' 0.05 `.' 0.1 ` ' 1
```

It can be seen that the treatment effect from the meta-estimate of -10.4810 is statistically significant with p-value < 0.0001, which indicated that the new drug significantly reduced blood pressure. This coincides with the pooled multi-center analysis in Section 1.4.2.2.

1.5 Summary and Recommendations for Further Reading

In this chapter, we introduced the reader to the R system, its installation, and its related packages. We illustrated the use of R for data simulation and manipulation, statistical graphics and statistical modeling by simulating data from a simple multi-center study.

For further reading to gain more familiar with the R system, we recommend:

- **R fundamentals to *S* languages**: Two books from John Chambers (Chambers (1998) and Chambers (2008)) are excellent references to understand the R language and its programming structures.

- **R graphics:** Besides Sarkar's book (Sarkar (2008)) on *lattice*, we also recommend Paul Murrell's book (Murrell (2005)).

- **Statistical data analysis using R:** We recommend Faraway's two books published in 2004 (Faraway (2004)) and 2006 (Faraway (2006)) which are excellent books using R for statistical modelling. Everitt and Hothorn's book (Everitt and Hothorn (2006)) on statistical data analysis using R is another excellent book we used in the classroom which interested students.

- **Statistical computing:** Maria Rizzo's book on statistical computing with R (Rizzo (2008)) is excellent.

- **Books for light reading:** There is a series of books in the bookstores which are written in very non-statistical fashion for readers to get familiar with R. We recommend Kabacoff (2011) which is a R language tutorial with focus on step-by-step practical problem solving, Gardener

(2012) which is written for users and data analysts with/without R knowledge, and Adler (2012) which covers every aspect of R and is an excellent reference book for R.

- **R online documentations:** We emphasize again that there are many free online books, manuals, journals and others to be downloaded from R homepage at "Documentation".

Chapter 2

Research Protocol for Meta-Analyses

2.1 Introduction

In this book, we present numerous examples of detailed meta-analysis in many areas of application using features of R. In doing so, with the exception of having access to patient level data in one chapter, we used summary data for a set of studies to be combined already meta-analyzed and reported in the literature. In presenting statistical details and results of our meta-analyses, we identified the research questions to which the meta-analyses appearing in the literature were directed. So we did not start by specifying a research question of interest, then perform searches of databases such as PUBMED, MEDLINE, PsycARTICLES or ERIC and identify the totality of studies that could provide summary information relative to the question, obtain publications of the studies, and then abstract the summary data to be synthesized.

In actual practice, if one were to have a question that a meta-analysis could possibly answer, the first and most important step is to write a protocol under which the totality of the meta-analysis inquiry as a scientific research effort would be conducted. The purpose of this chapter is to inform the reader of this most important exercise, briefly outline the steps involved in writing a meta-analysis protocol, and point the reader to publications that provide much detail and guidance in writing the protocol for a meta-analysis.

2.2 Defining the Research Objective

In developing a protocol for a clinical trial of a new drug, the first step is to formulate the objective or question that the trial seeks to answer as seen in Chapter 6 of Peace and Chen (2010). Beginning with a well-defined question as the first step in developing a protocol for a meta-analysis is of no less importance than beginning development of a protocol for a new drug with a well-defined question or objective. Some would argue that it may be more important as the opportunity for injecting bias may be greater.

As an example, suppose we were interested performing a meta-analysis based upon published studies of the following objective:

Objective: To assess the overall evidence of the effectiveness of calcium-channel blockers in the treatment of mild-to-moderate hypertension.

There are elements of the objective statement that are well defined; i.e. the drug class and the disease. However, searching the literature for mild-to-moderate hypertension may lead to publications that vary according to what is considered mild-to-moderate. So there is a need to specify

1. what is meant by mild-to-moderate. What is considered as normal blood pressure has changed over the years. So searching the literature for mild-to-moderate hypertension may identify older published studies where mild-to-moderate hypertension has a range of blood pressure that is shifted to the right of that in more recent studies. In addition, no mention is made of:

2. the effectiveness measure or outcome (and how assessed),

3. the type of control group,

4. study characteristics such as (a) type of design (parallel, crossover), (b) method of assignment (e.g. balanced random assignment) of patients to drug and control groups, (c) other measures to guard against bias (e.g. double-blinded),

5. type of patient (e.g. age range, race or ethnicity, gender, concomitant disease, etc.), or perhaps

6. length of study.

These six items essentially define parameters that govern the search for studies to be included in the meta-analysis to address the question or objective. Their importance relative to the objective statement is discussed in the following section of the protocol.

2.3 Criteria for Identifying Studies to Include in the Meta-Analysis

2.3.1 Clarifying the Disease under Study (What is meant by mild-to-moderate?)

What is considered as normal blood pressure has changed over the years (and thus so has what is considered as mild-to-moderate hypertension). For many years, the American Heart Association considered normal blood pressure for adults to be systolic blood pressure less than 140 mmHG and diastolic blood pressure less than 90 mmHG. More recently, the National Heart, Lung, and Blood Institute (NHLBI) in Bethesda, Maryland released new clinical guidelines for normal blood pressure in adults. They considered normal blood pressure in adults to be systolic less than 120 and diastolic to be less than 80. Over about a 20 year period, the definition of normal tension dropped by 20 mmHG systolic and 10 mmHG diastolic blood pressures. Hypertensive patients who entered trials per the AHA definition of normal blood pressure are likely to have blood pressure at baseline greater than that of patients who entered trials per the NHLBI.

After review of the references obtained, the meta-analysis researcher may wish to revise the objective, search for studies of hypertension and not restrict the search to mild-to-moderate hypertension.

2.3.2 The Effectiveness Measure or Outcome

In clinical trials of hypertension, the primary endpoint or effectiveness measure is change in diastolic blood pressure (DBP), where change in DBP is DBP after beginning treatment minus DBP just before beginning treatment (baseline). Systolic blood pressure (SBP) is measured and analyzed but is not considered primary. Since blood pressure varies with position (sitting, standing or supine) of the patient and with the method of assessment (digital recorder or sphygmomanometer) this information should be included as search parameters. Some trials may also report the proportion of patients in each treatment group who became normotensive. Older publications may include reports of change in mean arterial pressure (MAP), which is a weighted average of DBP and SBP. The point is that to synthesize results across trials, the same effectiveness measure must be determinable from each trial.

2.3.3 The Type of Control Group

Efficacy of a drug from a clinical trial is assessed relative to a control group. If the control is a matching placebo (negative control) then efficacy is viewed as direct efficacy. If the comparison of drug to placebo is statistically significant at some pre-specified small false positive rate, then direct evidence of efficacy would have been demonstrated. If the control is another drug (positive control), then the comparison of drug to the positive control provides a measure of the extent to which the drug is efficacious relative to the positive control. If positive control was already regulatory approved as efficacious, the difference between the drug and the positive control being small enough to conclude that drug was equivalent to the positive control supports indirect efficacy of the drug. There are other issues here relative to the comparability of the trial population to the population in which the efficacy of the positive control was established. But it should be clear that in identifying a group of studies for meta-analysis of a specific drug, studies included should contain both the drug group and the same control group.

2.3.4 Study Characteristics

Study characteristics are important in searching for studies that may be synthesized to address the objective of the meta-analysis. These include (a) the type of experimental design, such as whether it is crossover (each patient serves as his/ her own control) or parallel; (b) whether patients are randomly assigned to the treatment and control groups in balanced (equal numbers of patients to each group) or imbalanced (such as twice as many patients randomly assigned to the treatment group as to the control group) or whether randomization is in blocks to ensure balance across time of entry; (c) whether patients are stratified on prognostic factors prior to randomization; and (d) measures taken to eliminate or minimize bias (such as double-blinded: both investigational site personnel and patients are blinded as to identification of the intervention groups) or preserving blinding and preservation of the Type I error if group sequential analyses are performed in the study.

2.3.5 Type of Patient

Patient characteristics such as age, race or ethnicity, gender, whether patients in the studies are in or out of hospital during the treatment period, the existence of concurrent disease other than the one being treated by the new drug, and whether patients are permitted to take concomitant medications for the concurrent diseases all help to identify the type of patient in the inferenced population from the individual studies. Synthesizing studies that share common patient characteristics ensures that inference from the meta-analysis is to the same inferenced population. It is advisable for the researcher to abstract summary measures (e.g. mean, St.Dev. etc.) by treatment group for subgroups induced by the patient characteristics. The researcher could then address the extent to which inference to the general population extended to subgroups.

2.3.6 Length of Study

The length of the treatment period of the study is important in the study of hypertension (as well as in the study of many other diseases). Change in blood pressure from a study of say 1 month of treatment is different than blood pressure from a study of 6 months' duration.

2.4 Searching for and Collecting the Studies

There are many databases that may be searched for a particular meta-analysis. More popular ones are: PubMed (MEDLINE), Embase, Web of Science (Science Citation Index), ClinicalTrials.gov and the Cochrane Central Register of Controlled Trials. PubMed contains more than 22 million citations for biomedical literature from MEDLINE (`www.ncbi.nlm.nih.gov/pubmed`). MEDLINE is the largest component of PubMed as pointed out in Katcher (2006).

Embase contains more than 25 million indexed records and over 7,600 currently indexed peer-reviewed journals. Embase is a highly versatile, multipurpose and up-to-date database covering the most important international biomedical literature from 1947 to the present day (`http://www.embase.com/info/what-embase`).

Web of Science (Science Citation Index) indexes 6,000 key science journals since 1900. One can search by author, keywords, organization and cited reference (`https://libraries.ucsd.edu/info/resources/web-science-science-citation-index`).

`ClinicalTrials.gov` lists 137,011 studies with locations in all 50 states and in 182 countries (`http://www.clinicaltrials.gov/`). Using the search function located on the home page, we found 167 studies when searching for mild-to-moderate hypertension and 4877 studies were found when dropping mild-to-moderate and searching for hypertension.

The Cochrane Collaboration is an international network of over 28,000 dedicated people from more than 100 countries. They work together to help healthcare providers, policy-makers, patients, their advocates and care givers make well-informed decisions about health care, by preparing, updating, and promoting the accessibility of Cochrane Reviews - numbering over 5,000 and published online in the Cochrane Database of Systematic Reviews, part of The Cochrane Library. They also prepare the largest collection of records of randomized controlled trials in the world, called CENTRAL, which is published as part of The Cochrane Library. Their work is recognized internationally as the benchmark for high quality information about the effectiveness of health care (`http://www.cochrane.org/about-us`).

Chapters 6 and 7 of the Cochrane Handbook are particularly helpful in outlining and explaining the search and selection of studies (`http://www.cochrane.org/training/cochrane-handbook`).

The criteria for identifying studies to include in the meta-analysis are synonymous to the Inclusion/ Exclusion Criteria of a clinical trial protocol. Inclusion means the researcher decides which studies to keep for the meta-analysis. Exclusion means the researcher decides which studies not to keep. For a clinical trial protocol, inclusion/ exclusion criteria apply at the patient level. Inclusion/ exclusion criteria for meta-analysis apply at the study level.

Chapter 5 of the Cochrane Handbook (`http://www.mrc-bsu.cam.ac.uk/cochrane/handbook/`) uses the acronym PICO (Participants, Interventions, Comparisons and Outcomes) as a pneumonic to remind the researcher of the need for aliasing the question with essential components. The question, PICO and additional specifications of types of studies that will be included form the basis of the pre-specified eligibility criteria for the review.

Many other databases are available for searching. In addition to those noted above, the Countway Library of Medicine: An Alliance of the Boston Medical Library and Harvard Medical School (`http://hms.harvard.libguides.com/meta-analysis`), lists databases useful to biologists, nurses, cognitive and behavioral therapies researchers, reproductive and population issues researchers, researchers in community related and interpersonal issues, as well as other areas:

- **BIOSIS Previews**: Primarily useful to biologists, but also contains lots of meetings and some medical journals;
- **CINAHL**: Primarily contains information on nursing; an excellent source for issues in patient care;
- **PsycINFO**: Covers cognitive and behavioral therapies;
- **POPLINE**: Covers reproductive and population issues (`http://www.popline.org/`);
- **LILACS**: Contains health science literature published by Latin American and Caribbean authors (`http://bases.bireme.br/`);

- **African Index Medicus**: An index to African health literature and information sources at http://indexmedicus.afro.who.int/;
- **Other Regional WHO Databases**: Includes South-East Asia and Western Pacific regional databases at http://www.who.int/library/databases/en/;
- **Sociological Abstracts**: The primary index for sociological literature; may be useful for community-related studies or interpersonal issues.

The above databases for which the URL does not appear may be accessed with permission via Bain at http://hms.harvard.libguides.com/meta-analysis.

A database in the area of education is:

- **ERIC**: World's largest digital library of education literature; contains bibliographic records of education literature, plus a growing collection of full text (http://www.eric.ed.gov/),

and another in psychological areas is:

- **PsycARTICLES**: a database of full-text articles from journals published by the American Psychological Association, the APA Educational Publishing Foundation, the Canadian Psychological Association, and Hogrefe & Huber at http://www.csa.com/factsheets/psycarticles-set-c.php.

The databases listed represent a start for researchers in the areas identified. Researchers in other areas of meta-analysis application may identify other databases by searching the WWW and/ or making use of university libraries.

2.5 Data Abstraction and Extraction

The researcher should design a data extraction form (DAF) that is clear and unambiguous. It will be used to extract and record the data from studies that will be synthesized to address the objective of the meta-analysis (`http://ph.cochrane.org/sites/ph.cochrane.org/files/uploads/Unit_Seven.pdf`). Synthesis of the individual study findings proceeds easier from the DAF than working directly from the publication to analysis file creation. The DAF with extracted data creates a documentation record that can be used in a quality assurance process, or used by future researchers who may wish to update meta-analysis findings as more studies become available.

Reports of studies may vary in terms of the summary measures (e.g. means versus medians, standard deviations versus standard errors, etc.) reported and level of study detail. Meta-analysis researchers may need to contact the authors of the studies for any additional study details. In addition, researchers may find more than one report of the same study. Data from all reports should be abstracted and referenced on the DAF, but the researcher must determine which report is most accurate with respect to the number of patients and summary statistics. Again, the researcher may need to contact the authors to determine which report provides the appropriate summary measures to use for their meta-analysis.

It is good practice for researchers to pilot the DAF on a small group of studies to ensure that it captures all information required for their meta-analysis. If multiple reviewers and data extractors differ, every effort should be made to explain any differences among extractors and arrive at a consensus.

What to include on the DAF is guided primarily by the criteria for identifying studies to include in the meta-analysis. That is, the disease under study; the effectiveness measures or outcomes; the type of control group; study characteristics; type of patient and length of study.

The researcher will find Chapter 7: Selecting studies and collecting data, of the Cochrane Handbook, helpful (`http://www.cochrane.org/handbook/chapter-7-selecting-studies-and-collecting-data`). In particular, sections 7.5: Data collection forms, 7.6: Extracting data from reports and 7.7: Extracting study results and converting to the desired format provide guidance on data abstraction and extraction.

2.6 Meta-Analysis Methods

The meta-analysis methods section of the protocol will be guided by the objective, the type of data to be synthesized and the statistical methods appropriate for the data collected and the design of the study. This section should be written before undertaking searches for appropriate studies. It is important to address how heterogeneity of summary measures across studies will be addressed.

As is the case in writing the data analysis section of a protocol, the meta-analysis methods section may need to be modified based upon peculiarities found among studies identified in the search and data abstracted therefrom.

Chapter 9: Analyzing data and undertaking meta-analyses (edited by Deeks JI, Higgins JPT, Altman DG on behalf of the Cochrane Statistical Methods Group), from the Cochrane Collaboration Handbook (`http://www.cochrane.org/handbook`), is helpful to researchers in developing the meta-analysis methods section.

Of course meta-analysis methods (using R) are primarily the subject of this book. The researcher is encouraged to review chapters 3 through 9 for help in identifying methods appropriate for various summary data.

2.7 Results

We recommend that researchers produce stand alone reports of their meta-analysis research efforts. The outline of such a report would follow the protocol contents outline but may include appendices to make the report standalone. The report would include: an Abstract or Executive Summary, Objectives, Study Population, Locating (Searching for) Studies, Screening and Evaluation Methods (which includes Inclusion/Exclusion Criteria, Study Characteristics), Data Abstraction and Extraction, Meta-Analysis Methods, Results, Summary and Discussion, Conclusions, and Appendices.

Readers should view the results from the numerous meta-analyses in chapters 3-9 of this book for specificity of output (results), including graphical displays of effect sizes, assessment of heterogeneity and bias. The meta-analysis report plays the same role for the meta-analysis protocol as the clinical study report for a clinical trial protocol.

The meta-analysis report becomes the single best source of documentation of the meta-analysis research as a process. Once the report is developed, articles for publication may be developed.

2.8 Summary and Discussion

This chapter called attention to the importance of writing a protocol as the first step in a meta-analysis. After an initial introduction, we noted that a meta-analysis protocol (i.e. plan of study) would contain sections with content related to: **Defining the Research Objective, Criteria for Identifying Studies to include in the Meta-Analysis, Searching for and Collecting the Studies, Data Abstraction, Meta-Analysis Methods** and **Results**.

The section on Criteria for Identifying Studies to include in the Meta-Analysis had six subsections for further clarity. These are: Clarifying the disease under study, The effectiveness measure or outcome, The type of control group, Study characteristics, Type of patient and Length of study.

Berman and Parker (2002) acknowledge that the totality of a meta-analysis resembles a conventional study, requiring a written protocol. They provide a structure for creating a meta-analysis protocol and list some guidelines for measuring the quality of papers that may provide summary information to be synthesized.

In addition, Chapter 4: Guide to the contents of a Cochrane protocol and review (edited by Higgins JPT, Green S) from the Cochrane Collaboration Handbook (`http://www.cochrane.org/handbook/chapter-4-guide-contents-cochrane-protocol-and-review`) is helpful to researchers in developing a meta-analysis protocol.

The report authored by West et al. (2002) for the Agency for Healthcare Research and Quality entitled "Systems to Rate the Strength of Scientific Evidence" is a must read. It recognizes the importance of developing a well-designed protocol to guide the totality of the meta-analysis inquiry as a scientific research effort. "Thus, **before** a research team conducts a systematic review, it develops a well-designed protocol that lists: (1) a focused study question, (2) a specific search strategy, including the databases to be searched, and how studies will be identified and selected for the review according to inclusion and exclusion criteria, (3) the types of data to be abstracted from each article, and (4) how the data will be synthesized, either as a text summary or as some type of quantitative aggregation or meta-analysis. These steps are taken to protect the work against various forms of unintended bias in the identification, selection, and use of published work in these reviews."

Further, the main sections of this chapter and subsections of section 2.3, pertain largely to medical questions or questions based on clinical trials. Section and subsection topics are applicable regardless of the application with few modifications. For example, subsection 2.3.1 Clarifying the Disease under Study in general would be Clarifying the Area of Application; 2.3.5 Type of Patients would be Specifying the Experimental, Sampling or Analysis Unit.

Regardless of the application, the researcher must first write a scientifically defensible protocol that will guide the totality of the meta-analysis inquiry as a scientific research effort. The protocol should include the sections: Defining the Research Objective, Criteria for Identifying Studies to include in the Meta-Analysis, Searching for and Collecting the Studies, Data Abstraction, Meta-Analysis Methods and Results. After writing the protocol, identifying data sources, and abstracting the data, the data may be meta-analyzed by methods that are largely independent of the application.

Chapter 3

Fixed-Effects and Random-Effects in Meta-Analysis

To any analyst performing a meta-analysis, the first terminology is probably fixed-effects versus random-effects models. Therefore to give readers an introductory and broad view of meta-analysis, we begin by presenting these models with limited details in this chapter along with the commonly used R packages of `rmeta` and `meta` using two datasets described in Section 3.1. Detailed descriptions of these models and their applications will be learned in future chapters.

The first dataset is the classical and famous data from Cochrane Collaboration logo that resulted from systematic reviews of the entire, pre-1980 clinical study literature of corticosteroid therapy in premature labor and its effect on neonatal death. The meta-analysis figure is part of the logo of the Cochrane Collaboration (`http://www.cochrane.org`). We present meta-analyses of this dataset using the R system. The response measure in this dataset is binary (death or alive).

The second dataset contains estimates of treatment effect from eight randomized controlled trials of the effectiveness of amlodipine as compared to placebo in improving work capacity in patients with angina. The response measure in this dataset is "work capacity" which is continuous.

In Section 3.2, we introduce fixed-effects and random-effects models used in meta-analysis where fixed-effects is the weighted mean method and random effects is the DerSimonian-Laird random-effects model implemented in R libraries `rmeta` (Author: Thomas Lumley from the Department of Biostatistics at the University of Washington, USA) and `meta` (Author: Guido Schwarzer from the Institute for Medical Biometry and Medical Informatics at the University Hospital Freiburg, Germany). The library `rmete` is used mainly for binary data whereas the library meta may be used for both binary and continuous data. In Section 3.3, we demonstrate how to use R and the R functionalities from both libraries to analyze the two datasets in this chapter. Discussion and recommendations appear in 3.5.

Note: to run the R programs in this chapter, readers should first install the following R packages: gdata to read the data, rmeta and meta to perform meta-analysis.

3.1 Two Datasets from Clinical Studies

3.1.1 Data for Cochrane Collaboration Logo: Binary Data

Data from seven randomized controlled trials conducted prior to 1980 of corticosteroid therapy in premature labor and its effect on neonatal death were meta-analyzed. These data are included in R meta-analysis library rmeta and are reproduced in Table 3.1 for easy reference. This data frame contains five columns. Column 1 contains the "name" as an identifier for the study. Column 2 contains the number ("ev.trt") of deaths among patients in the treated group. Column 3 contains the total number of patients ("n.trt") in the treated group. Column 4 contains the number of deaths ("ev.ctrl") in the control group. Column 5 contains the total number of patients ("n.ctrl") in the control group.

TABLE 3.1: Data for Cochrane Collaboration Logo.

name	ev.trt	n.trt	ev.ctrl	n.ctrl
Auckland	36	532	60	538
Block	1	69	5	61
Doran	4	81	11	63
Gamsu	14	131	20	137
Morrison	3	67	7	59
Papageorgiou	1	71	7	75
Tauesch	8	56	10	71

3.1.2 Clinical Studies on Amlodipine: Continuous Data

Eight randomized controlled trials of the effectiveness of the calcium channel blocker amlodipine as compared to placebo in improving work capacity in patients with angina are summarized in Table 3.2. These data are used in Li et al. (1994) to illustrate potential bias in meta-analysis. The data are reproduced further in Hartung et al. (2008). The change in work capacity is defined as the ratio of exercise time after the patient receives the intervention (i.e. drug or placebo) to the exercise time at baseline (before receiving the intervention). It is assumed that the logarithms of these ratios are normally distributed. Table 3.2 lists the observed sample size, mean and variance for both treatment and placebo groups. We meta-analyze these data to illustrate application of (meta-analysis) methods for continuous data.

TABLE 3.2: Angina Study Data

Protocol	nE	meanE	varE	nC	meanC	varC
154	46	0.2316	0.2254	48	-0.0027	0.0007
156	30	0.2811	0.1441	26	0.0270	0.1139
157	75	0.1894	0.1981	72	0.0443	0.4972
162	12	0.0930	0.1389	12	0.2277	0.0488
163	32	0.1622	0.0961	34	0.0056	0.0955
166	31	0.1837	0.1246	31	0.0943	0.1734
303	27	0.6612	0.7060	27	-0.0057	0.9891
306	46	0.1366	0.1211	47	-0.0057	0.1291

3.2 Fixed-Effects and Random-Effects Models in Meta-Analysis

As described in Wikipedia, "In statistics, a meta-analysis combines the results of several studies that address a set of related research hypotheses. This is normally done by identification of a common measure of *effect size*, which is modeled using a form of meta-regression. Resulting overall averages when controlling for study characteristics can be considered meta-effect sizes, which are more powerful estimates of the true effect size than those derived in a single study under a given single set of assumptions and conditions". We thus begin introducing this *effect size* in Section 3.2.1.

3.2.1 Hypotheses and Effect Size

The fundamental objective for conducting a clinical study of the efficacy of a new drug (D) in the treatment of some disease is to demonstrate that the new drug is effective in treating the disease. Translating into the statistical hypothesis framework, the objective becomes the alternative hypothesis in contrast to the null hypothesis of inefficacy given by:

$$H_0 : \text{Effect of D is no different from that of control (placebo = P)}$$
$$H_a : \text{Effect of D is better than that of P}$$

Treatment effect size is a comparative function of the efficacy response measure in each treatment group. The comparative function may be the difference in means if response is continuous, or the difference in proportions if response in dichotomous or binary. Other comparative functions of effect size for binary data are the log-odds ratio or relative risk. It is noted that the comparative function specifies an arithmetical order of the interventions; e.g. drug-control or drug/control. The treatment effect size is denoted by δ to be compatible with the notations used in Peace and Chen (2010). Then H_0 and H_a above become:

$$H_0 : \delta = 0$$
$$H_a : \delta > 0$$

For multiple randomized, controlled, efficacy studies of a drug, H_0 and H_a are the same for each study. Randomization of patients to treatment groups within studies and conducting the study in a blinded and quality manner ensures valid, unbiased estimates of treatment effect within studies.

Fundamentally a design-based analysis strategy is no different than a meta-analysis of the treatment effect estimates across the centers. That is, first compute the estimates of treatment effect $\hat{\delta}_i$ and the within variance $\hat{\sigma}_i^2$ of treatment effect at each study or center $i(i = 1, \cdots, K)$, and then meta-analyze the $\hat{\delta}_i$ across studies or centers.

To obtain an estimate of the overall efficacy of the drug across all studies and to provide an inference as to the statistical significance of the overall effect, the individual study estimates are meta-analyzed. There are typically two meta-analysis approaches in this direction with one as *fixed-effects* and the other as *random-effects*.

In fixed-effects meta-analysis, we assume that we have an estimate of *treatment effect* $\hat{\delta}_i$ and its (within) variability estimate $\hat{\sigma}_i^2$ from each clinical study i. Each $\hat{\delta}_i$ is an estimate of the underlying global overall effect of δ across all studies. To meta-analyze this set of $\hat{\delta}_i$ means that we combine them using some weighting scheme.

However, for the random-effects meta-analysis model, we assume that each $\hat{\delta}_i$ is an estimate of its own underlying true effect δ_i which is one realization from the overall global effect δ. Therefore, the random-effects meta-analysis model can incorporate both within-study variability and between-study variability - which may be an important source of heterogeneity in multiple studies.

3.2.2 Fixed-Effects Meta-Analysis Model: The Weighted-Average

3.2.2.1 Fixed-Effects Model

The underlying assumption for the fixed-effects model is that all studies in the meta-analysis share a common (true) overall effect size δ with same impacts from all other risk factors. With that assumption, the true effect size is the same (and therefore the name of *fixed-effects*) in all the studies. In this fixed-effects model, each observed effect size $\hat{\delta}_i$ could vary among studies because of the random errors from each study and is assumed to be an estimate of the underlying global overall effect δ.

Under the fixed-effects model we assume that all factors that could influence the effect size are the same in all the studies, and that

$$\hat{\delta}_i = \delta + \epsilon_i \tag{3.1}$$

where ϵ_i is assumed to be normally distributed by $N(0, \hat{\sigma}_i^2)$. That is

$$\hat{\delta}_i \sim N(\delta, \hat{\sigma}_i^2) \tag{3.2}$$

The global δ is then estimated by combining the individual estimates by some weighting scheme in order to obtain the most precise estimate of the global effect. That is, we weight $\hat{\delta}_i$ for each study i with an appropriate weight w_i, then compute the weighted mean or pooled estimate $\hat{\delta}$ of treatment effect as well as its variance $\hat{\sigma}^2$, where

$$\hat{\delta} = \sum_{i=1}^{K} w_i \hat{\delta}_i \tag{3.3}$$

$$\hat{\sigma}^2 = Var(\hat{\delta}) = \sum_{i=1}^{K} w_i^2 \hat{\sigma}_i^2 (\text{under independence of the K studies}) \tag{3.4}$$

Using the weighted mean in equation 3.3 and its variance in equation 3.4, an approximate 95% confidence interval (CI) for δ is:

$$\hat{\delta} \pm 1.96 \times \sqrt{\hat{\sigma}^2} \tag{3.5}$$

In addition, we may formulate a t-type of test as:

$$T = \frac{\hat{\delta} - \delta}{\sqrt{\hat{\sigma}^2}} \tag{3.6}$$

to be used to test $H_0 : \delta = 0$. Based on the test statistic in equation 3.6, we construct confidence intervals on the overall global effect of δ in the usual manner.

3.2.2.2 The Weighting Schemes

The weighted mean in equation (3.3), requires $\sum_{i=1}^{K} w_i = 1$. Typical choices of w_i are:

1. Weighting by the number of studies as

$$w_i = \frac{1}{K} \tag{3.7}$$

   where K is the number of studies(fixed);

2. Weighting by the number of patients in each study as:

$$w_i = \frac{N_i}{N} \tag{3.8}$$

where N_i is the number of patients in study i, and N is the total number of patients as $N = \sum_{i=1}^{K} N_i$;

3. Weighting by the number of patients from each study and each treatment as:

$$w_i = \frac{N_{iD}N_{iP}}{N_{iD} + N_{iP}} \times \frac{1}{w} \tag{3.9}$$

where $w = \sum_{i=1}^{K} w_i$ and N_{iD} and N_{iP} are the numbers of patients in the new drug treatment (D) and Placebo (P) groups respectively at study i;

4. Weighting by the inverse variance

$$w_i = \frac{1}{\hat{\sigma}_i^2} \times \frac{1}{w} \tag{3.10}$$

where $w = \sum_{i=1}^{K} w_i$.

The weighting scheme 1 in equation 3.7 yields the unweighted mean or arithmetic average of the estimates of treatment effect across studies.

The weighting scheme 2 in equation 3.8 yields the average of the estimates of treatment effect across studies weighted according to the number of patients at each study. Note that the weighting scheme 2 in equation 3.8 reduces to weight scheme 1 in equation 3.7 if there is balance across studies.

The weighting scheme 3 in equation 3.9 yields the average of the estimates of treatment effect across studies weighted to allow treatment group imbalance at each study. Note that scheme 3 in equation 3.9 reduces to scheme 2 in equation 3.8 if treatment groups are balanced across studies.

The weighting scheme 4 in equation 3.10 yields the average of the estimates of treatment effect across studies weighting the estimates inversely to their variance; this is used in almost all fixed-effects models and we will use this weighting hereafter. Note that scheme 4 in equation 3.10 reduces to scheme 1 in equation 3.7 if the $\hat{\sigma}_i^2$ are the same (true homogeneity) across studies.

It should be noted that for dichotomous response data, the data at each study may be summarized by a two-by-two table with responders versus non-responders as columns and treatment groups as rows. Let O_i denote the number of responders in the pivotal cell of the two-by-two table at each study, and $E(O_i)$ and $Var(O_i)$ denote the expected value and variance of O_i, respectively, computed from the hypergeometric distribution. The square of equation 3.6 becomes the Mantel-Haenszel statistic (unadjusted for lack of continuity) proposed by Mantel and Haenszel (1959) for addressing association between treatment and response across studies. For this reason, the weighted mean estimate in 3.3 with its variance in 3.4 using weighting scheme 4 is implemented in R library `rmeta` as function `meta.MH` for "*Fixed effects (Mantel-Haenszel) meta-analysis*". This R library is created by Professor Thomas Lumley at the University of Washington with functions for simple fixed and random-effects meta-analysis for two-sample comparisons and cumulative meta-analyses as well as drawing standard summary plots, funnel plots, and computing summaries and tests for association and heterogeneity.

3.2.3 Random-Effects Meta-Analysis Model: DerSimonian-Laird

3.2.3.1 Random-Effects Model

When meta-analyzing effect sizes from different studies (such as separate clinical trials), the fundamental assumption in the fixed-effects model that the true effect size is the same for all studies may be impractical. When we attempt to synthesize a group of studies with a meta-analysis, we expect that these studies have enough in common to combine the information for statistical inference, but it would be impractical to require that these studies have identical true effect size.

The random-effects meta-analysis model assumes the treatment effect $\hat{\delta}_{iR}$ from each study i is an estimate of its own underlying true treatment effect δ_{iR} with variance σ_i^2, and further that the δ_{iR} from all the K studies follow some overall global distribution denoted by $N(\delta, \tau^2)$. This random-effects meta model can be written as:

$$\begin{aligned} \hat{\delta}_{iR} &\sim N(\delta_{iR}, \sigma_i^2) \\ \delta_{iR} &\sim N(\delta, \tau^2) \end{aligned} \quad (3.11)$$

This random-effects model can be described as an extension of the fixed-effects model in equation 3.1 as:

$$\hat{\delta}_{iR} = \delta + \nu_i + \epsilon_i \quad (3.12)$$

where $\nu_i \sim N(0, \tau^2)$ describes the between-center variation.

We make the assumption that ν_i and ϵ_i are independent and therefore, the random-effects model in equation 3.11 can be re-written as:

$$\hat{\delta}_{iR} \sim N(\delta, \sigma_i^2 + \tau^2) \quad (3.13)$$

In this formulation, the extra parameter τ^2 represents the between-study variability around the underlying global treatment effect δ. It is easy to show in this formulation that the global δ is also estimated by the weighted mean similar to the fixed-effects meta-model as given in equation 3.3 as:

$$\hat{\delta}_R = \frac{\sum_{i=1}^K w_{iR}\hat{\delta}_{iR}}{\sum_{i=1}^K w_{iR}} \quad (3.14)$$

with standard error estimated as:

$$se\left(\hat{\delta}_R\right) = \sqrt{\frac{1}{\sum_{i=1}^K w_{iR}}} \quad (3.15)$$

where the weights now are given by:

$$\hat{w}_{iR} = \frac{1}{\hat{\sigma}_i^2 + \hat{\tau}^2} \quad (3.16)$$

$$se\left(\hat{\delta}_R\right) = \sqrt{\frac{1}{\sum_{i=1}^K w_{iR}}} \quad (3.17)$$

Therefore, a 95% CI may be formulated to provide statistical inference similar to the fixed-effects model.

There are several methods to estimate the $\hat{\tau}^2$. The most commonly used estimate is from DerSimonian and Laird (1986) and is derived using the method of moments (which does not involve iterative search algorithms as do likelihood-based ones). Parenthetically, we note that the DerSimonian-Laird procedure is commonly referred to as the Cochran-DerSimonian-Laird procedure due to the work Cochran did in the mid-1950s on combining data from a series of experiments. This estimate is given as:

$$\hat{\tau}^2 = \frac{Q - (K-1)}{U} \tag{3.18}$$

if $Q > K - 1$, otherwise, $\hat{\tau}^2 = 0$ where

$$Q = \sum_{i=1}^{K} w_i(\hat{\delta}_i - \hat{\delta})^2 \tag{3.19}$$

$$U = \sum_{i=1}^{K} w_i - \frac{\sum_{i=1}^{K} w_i^2}{\sum_{i=1}^{K} w_i} \tag{3.20}$$

Note that the statistic Q is used for testing the statistical significance of heterogeneity across studies. This random-effects meta-model is implemented in the R library `rmeta` as function `meta.DSL` for "*Random effects (DerSimonian-Laird) meta-analysis*". It is also implemented as `metabin` and `metacont` in library `meta`.

Therefore, the random-effects meta-analysis model can incorporate both within-study and between-study variability which may be an important source of heterogeneity for meta-analysis. In this sense, the random-effects meta-analysis model is more conservative since $w_{iR} \leq w_i$ which leads to

$$se(\hat{\delta}_R) = \sqrt{\frac{1}{\sum_{i=1}^{K} w_{iR}}} \geq \sqrt{\frac{1}{\sum_{i=1}^{K} w_i}} = se(\hat{\delta}). \tag{3.21}$$

3.2.3.2 Derivation of DerSimonian-Laird Estimator of τ^2

The derivation of DerSimonian-Laird estimator of τ^2 in equation (3.18) is based on the method of moments by equating the sample statistic of Q to the corresponding expected value.

To emphasize here again that the only difference between the fixed-effects and the random-effects is the weighting factors in the weighted-average where in the random-effects $\hat{w}_{iR} = \frac{1}{\hat{\sigma}_i^2 + \hat{\tau}^2}$ and in the fixed-effects $\hat{w}_i = \frac{1}{\hat{\sigma}_i^2}$. Corresponding to these weighting factors, the meta-estimators are $\hat{\delta}_R = \frac{\sum_{i=1}^{K} w_{iR}\hat{\delta}_{iR}}{\sum_{i=1}^{K} w_{iR}}$ for random-effects and $\hat{\delta} = \frac{\sum_{i=1}^{K} w_i\hat{\delta}_i}{\sum_{i=1}^{K} w_i}$ for fixed-effects.

It can be shown that both estimators of $\hat{\delta}^*$ and $\hat{\delta}$ are unbiased with expected value of δ. The variances are

$$var\left(\hat{\delta}\right) = \frac{1}{\sum_{i=1}^{K} w_i} \tag{3.22}$$

$$var\left(\hat{\delta}_R\right) = \frac{1}{\sum_{i=1}^{K} w_{iR}} \tag{3.23}$$

With these facts, we can now derive the DerSimonian-Laird estimator. Let's first decompose the Q as

$$\begin{aligned} Q &= \sum_{i=1}^{K} w_i(\hat{\delta}_i - \hat{\delta})^2 = \sum_{i=1}^{K} w_i \left[(\hat{\delta}_i - \delta) - (\hat{\delta} - \delta)\right]^2 \\ &= \sum_{i=1}^{K} w_i(\hat{\delta}_i - \delta)^2 - 2\sum_{i=1}^{K} w_i(\hat{\delta}_i - \delta)(\hat{\delta} - \delta) + \sum_{i=1}^{K} w_i(\hat{\delta} - \delta)^2 \end{aligned} \tag{3.24}$$

Therefore the expected values of Q under **random-effects model** in equation (3.11) can be shown as follows:

$$\begin{aligned} E(Q) &= \sum_{i=1}^{K} w_i E(\hat{\delta}_i - \delta)^2 - \left(\sum_{i=1}^{K} w_i\right) E(\hat{\delta} - \delta)^2 \\ &= \sum_{i=1}^{K} w_i var(\hat{\delta}_i) - \left(\sum_{i=1}^{K} w_i\right) var(\hat{\delta}) \\ &= \sum_{i=1}^{K} w_i var(\hat{\delta}_i) - \left(\sum_{i=1}^{K} w_i\right) var\left[\frac{\sum_{i=1}^{K} w_i\hat{\delta}_i}{\sum_{i=1}^{K} w_i}\right] \\ &= \sum_{i=1}^{K} w_i var(\hat{\delta}_i) - \left(\sum_{i=1}^{K} w_i\right) \frac{\sum_{i=1}^{K} w_i^2 var\left(\hat{\delta}_i\right)}{\left(\sum_{i=1}^{K} w_i\right)^2} \\ &= \sum_{i=1}^{K} w_i(w_i^{-1} + \tau^2) - \left(\sum_{i=1}^{K} w_i\right) \frac{\sum_{i=1}^{K} w_i^2(w_i^{-1} + \tau^2)}{\left(\sum_{i=1}^{K} w_i\right)^2} \\ &= \sum_{i=1}^{K} w_i(w_i^{-1} + \tau^2) - \left(\sum_{i=1}^{K} w_i\right) \left[\frac{1}{\sum_{i=1}^{K} w_i} + \frac{\tau^2 \sum_{i=1}^{K} w_i^2}{\left(\sum_{i=1}^{K} w_i\right)^2}\right] \\ &= (K-1) + \tau^2 \left[\sum_{i=1}^{K} w_i - \frac{\sum_{i=1}^{K} w_i^2}{\sum_{i=1}^{K} w_i}\right] \end{aligned} \tag{3.25}$$

For the method of moments, let $E(Q) \approx Q$ to estimate the τ^2 as

$$\hat{\tau}^2 = \frac{Q - (K-1)}{\sum_{i=1}^K w_i - \frac{\sum_{i=1}^K w_i^2}{\sum_{i=1}^K w_i}} \tag{3.26}$$

which is the well-known DerSimonian-Laird method of moments for τ^2 in equation (3.18). Notice that the estimated variance $\hat{\tau}^2$ can be less than zero even though the true variance of τ^2 can never be. This happens when $Q < df = K - 1$ and when this happens, the estimated $\hat{\tau}^2$ is set to zero.

3.2.4 Publication Bias

Publication bias is sometimes referred to as selection bias. In meta-analysis, the studies selected to be included are vital to the inferential conclusion. Publication bias could arise when only positive studies (those that demonstrate statistical significance or if not statistically significant don't reflect qualitative interaction) of a drug are published. Therefore even though all published studies of a drug for the treatment of some disease may be selected for a meta-analysis, the resulting inferential results may be biased (may over estimate the efficacy of the drug). The bias may be particularly significant when meta-analyses are conducted or are sponsored by a group with a vested interest in the results.

In meta-analysis, Begg's *funnel plot* or Egger's plot is used to graphically display the existence of publication bias. Statistical tests for publication bias are usually based on the fact that clinical studies with small sample sizes (and therefore large variances) may be more prone to publication bias in contrast to large clinical studies. Therefore, when estimates from all studies are plotted against their variances (sample size), a symmetrical funnel should be seen when there is no publication bias, while a skewed asymmetrical funnel is a signal of potential publication bias. We illustrate this funnel plot along with the data analysis using the R system.

3.3 Data Analysis in R

3.3.1 Meta-Analysis for Cochrane Collaboration Logo

We illustrate meta-analysis using R package `rmeta`. First we access the "Cochrane" data and load it into R as:

```
> # Load the data
> data(cochrane)
> # print it
> cochrane
```

```
         name ev.trt n.trt ev.ctrl n.ctrl
1    Auckland     36   532      60    538
2       Block      1    69       5     61
3       Doran      4    81      11     63
4       Gamsu     14   131      20    137
5    Morrison      3    67       7     59
6 Papageorgiou     1    71       7     75
7     Tauesch      8    56      10     71
```

This gives the data in Table 3.1.

3.3.1.1 Fitting the Fixed-Effects Model

With this dataframe, we first fit the fixed-effects model as described in Section 3.2.2 using the R function `meta.MH` to compute the individual odds ratios or relative risks, the Mantel-Haenszel weighted mean estimate and Woolf's test for heterogeneity. The R implementation is illustrated by the following R code chunk:

```
> # Fit the fixed-effects model
> steroid = meta.MH(n.trt, n.ctrl, ev.trt, ev.ctrl,
                    names=name, data=cochrane)
> # Print the model fit
> summary(steroid)
```

```
Fixed effects ( Mantel-Haenszel ) meta-analysis
Call:meta.MH(ntrt=n.trt,nctrl=n.ctrl,ptrt=ev.trt,
    pctrl = ev.ctrl, names = name, data = cochrane)
------------------------------------
               OR (lower  95% upper)
Auckland      0.58    0.38        0.89
Block         0.16    0.02        1.45
Doran         0.25    0.07        0.81
Gamsu         0.70    0.34        1.45
Morrison      0.35    0.09        1.41
Papageorgiou 0.14    0.02        1.16
Tauesch       1.02    0.37        2.77
------------------------------------
Mantel-Haenszel OR =0.53 95% CI ( 0.39,0.73 )
Test for heterogeneity: X^2( 6 ) = 6.9 ( p-value 0.3303 )
```

It is observed from the model fit that the overall OR is 0.53 with 95% CI of (0.39, 0.73), indicating significant overall effect for steroid treatment in reducing neonatal death. However, if analyzed individually, in only two ("Auckland" and "Doran") of the seven studies was steroid treatment statistically significant. In addition, the χ^2 test for heterogeneity yielded a p-value of 0.3303 indicating non-statistically significant heterogeneity.

We could call the default function `plot` to plot the meta-analysis, but we can produce a more comprehensive figure for this analysis by calling the `forestplot` using the following R code chunk which gives Figure 3.1. This is the so-called "forest plot" in meta-analysis; i.e. a plot of the estimates and their associated 95% CIs for each study, as well as the global (summary or combined) estimate. The 95% CI intervals are the lines; the squares in the middle of the lines represent the point estimates. The global estimate or "Summary" is the diamond whose width is the associated 95% CI.

```
> # Create the ``tabletext" to include all the outputs
> tabletext = cbind(c("","Study",steroid$names,NA,"Summary"),
           c("Deaths","(Steroid)",cochrane$ev.trt,NA,NA),
           c("Deaths","(Placebo)",cochrane$ev.ctrl, NA,NA),
                  c("","OR",format(exp(steroid$logOR),digits=2),
```

```
                NA,format(exp(steroid$logMH),digits=2)))
> # Generate the CI
> mean   = c(NA,NA,steroid$logOR,NA,steroid$logMH)
> stderr = c(NA,NA,steroid$selogOR,NA,steroid$selogMH)
> l      = mean-1.96*stderr
> u      = mean+1.96*stderr
> # Call forestplot
> forestplot(tabletext,mean,l,u,zero=0,
       is.summary=c(TRUE,TRUE,rep(FALSE,8),TRUE),
  clip=c(log(0.1),log(2.5)), xlog=TRUE)
```

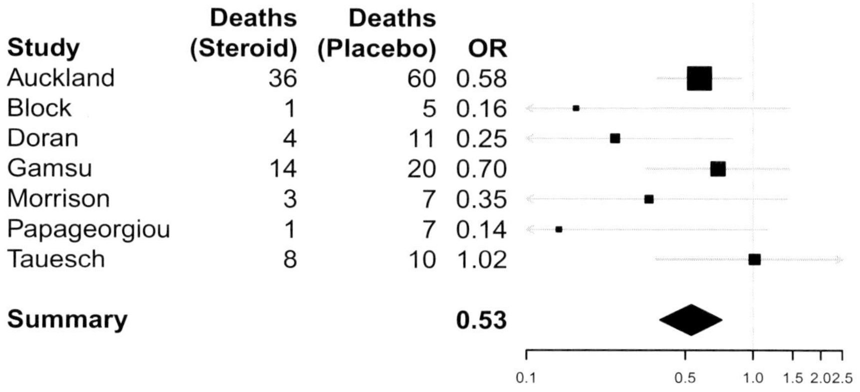

Study
Deaths (Steroid)
Deaths (Placebo)
OR
Auckland 36 60 0.58
Block 1 5 0.16
Doran 4 11 0.25
Gamsu 14 20 0.70
Morrison 3 7 0.35
Papageorgiou 1 7 0.14
Tauesch 8 10 1.02
Summary 0.53
0.1
0.5
1.0
1.5
2.0
2.5

FIGURE 3.1: `Forestplot` for Cochrane Data

3.3.1.2 Fitting the Random-Effects Model

Similarly, the random-effects model as described in Section 3.2.3 can be implemented using R function meta.DSL to compute the individual odds ratios or relative risks, the Mantel-Haenszel weighted mean estimate and Woolf's test for heterogeneity along with the estimate of the random-effects variance. The R implementation is illustrated by the following R code chunk:

```
> # Call the meta.DSL for calculations
> steroidDSL  = meta.DSL(n.trt,n.ctrl,ev.trt,ev.ctrl,
       names=name, data=cochrane)
> # Print the summary from meta.DSL
> summary(steroidDSL)

Random effects ( DerSimonian-Laird ) meta-analysis
Call: meta.DSL(ntrt= n.trt, nctrl = n.ctrl, ptrt = ev.trt,
    pctrl = ev.ctrl,names = name, data = cochrane)
------------------------------------
               OR (lower  95% upper)
Auckland     0.58     0.38      0.89
Block        0.16     0.02      1.45
Doran        0.25     0.07      0.81
Gamsu        0.70     0.34      1.45
Morrison     0.35     0.09      1.41
Papageorgiou 0.14     0.02      1.16
Tauesch      1.02     0.37      2.77
------------------------------------
SummaryOR= 0.53  95% CI ( 0.37,0.78 )
Test for heterogeneity: X^2( 6 ) = 6.86 ( p-value 0.334 )
Estimated random effects variance: 0.03
```

From the summary, we see that the estimated between-study variance = 0.03 and the global OR = 0.53 with 95% CI of (0.37, 0.78). Because of the estimated non zero between-study variance, the 95% CIs from individual studies and the one based on the global estimate are slightly wider than those from the fixed-effects meta-analysis - which is consistent with the theory described in Section 3.2.3. Both fixed-effects and random-effects models indicate a significant overall effect for steroid treatment in reducing neonatal death.

Similarly, the random-effects meta-analysis can be easily shown graphically in Figure 3.2 with the default `plot` setting. We encourage readers to use `forestplot` to reproduce this figure with different settings.

```
> plot(steroidDSL)
```

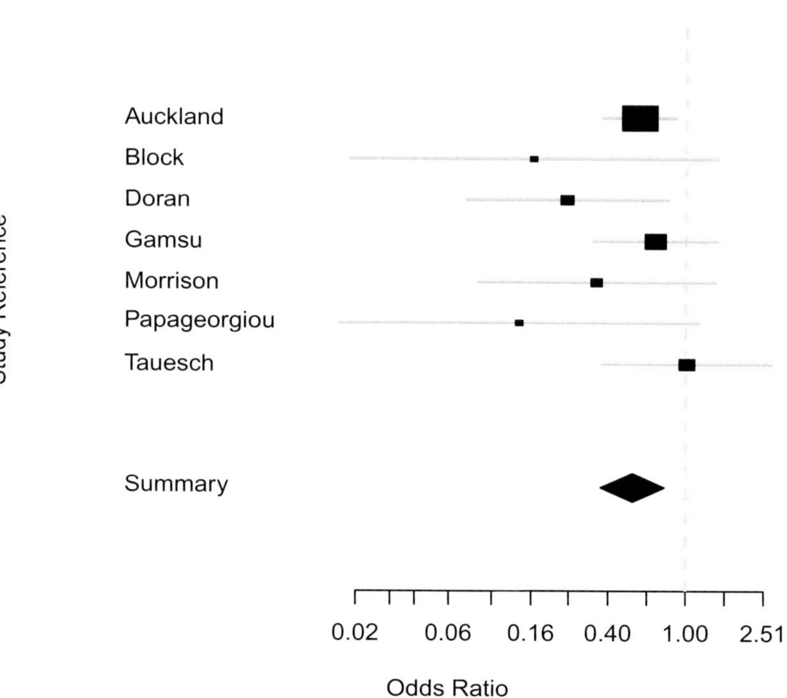

FIGURE 3.2: Forest Plot for the Cochran Trial with 95% CIs from Random-Effects Meta-Analysis

3.3.2 Analysis of Amlodipine Trial Data

3.3.2.1 Load the Library and Data

For this data, we illustrate the application of the R library `meta` for its functionalities in meta-analysis. We load the library as:

```
> library(meta)
```

The functions associated with this library may be seen using:

```
> library(help=meta)
```

This library may be used also for fixed- and random-effects meta-analysis. In addition, there are functions that can be used for tests of bias, and for producing forest and funnel plots. We load the data in Table 3.2 into R using R library `gdata` as follows:

```
> # Load the library
> require(gdata)
> # Get the data path
> datfile = "Your Data Path/dat4Meta.xls"
> # Call "read.xls" to read the Excel data sheet
> angina  = read.xls(datfile, sheet="Data_Angina",
             perl="c:/perl64/bin/perl.exe")
> # Print the data
> angina
```

```
  Protocol nE meanE   varE nC   meanC   varC
1      154 46 0.232 0.2254 48 -0.0027 0.0007
2      156 30 0.281 0.1441 26  0.0270 0.1139
3      157 75 0.189 0.1981 72  0.0443 0.4972
4      162 12 0.093 0.1389 12  0.2277 0.0488
5      163 32 0.162 0.0961 34  0.0056 0.0955
6      166 31 0.184 0.1246 31  0.0943 0.1734
7      303 27 0.661 0.7060 27 -0.0057 0.9891
8      306 46 0.137 0.1211 47 -0.0057 0.1291
```

We see that there are eight protocols or studies, each with the number of observations, mean and variance for treatment and control groups.

3.3.2.2 Fit the Fixed-Effects Model

This is a dataset with continuous response data and we use the `metacont` to model the data with the following R chunk:

```
> # Fit fixed-effect model
> fixed.angina = metacont(nE, meanE, sqrt(varE),
                          nC,meanC,sqrt(varC),
          data=angina,studlab=Protocol,comb.random=FALSE)
> # Print the fitted model
> fixed.angina

         MD             95%-CI %W(fixed)
154  0.2343  [ 0.0969; 0.372]     21.22
156  0.2541  [ 0.0663; 0.442]     11.35
157  0.1451  [-0.0464; 0.337]     10.92
162 -0.1347  [-0.3798; 0.110]      6.67
163  0.1566  [ 0.0072; 0.306]     17.94
166  0.0894  [-0.1028; 0.282]     10.85
303  0.6669  [ 0.1758; 1.158]      1.66
306  0.1423  [-0.0015; 0.286]     19.39

Number of studies combined: k=8

                       MD            95%-CI    z  p.value
Fixed effect model 0.162  [0.0986; 0.225] 5.01  <0.0001

Quantifying heterogeneity:
tau^2 = 0.0066; H = 1.33 [1; 2]; I^2 = 43.2% [0%; 74.9%]

Test of heterogeneity:
     Q d.f.  p.value
 12.33    7   0.0902

Details on meta-analytical method:
- Inverse variance method
```

From this fixed-effects model fitting, we note from the 95% CIs that amlodipine treatment is not statistically significant in four of the eight protocols. However, the overall effect of amlodipine from the fixed-effects model is 0.1619 with corresponding 95% CI of [0.0986; 0.2252] and p-value < 0.001 – indicating a statistically significant treatment effect. The test of heterogeneity gave a p-value of 0.09 from $Q = 12.33$ with degrees of freedom of 7 indicating that there is no strong evidence against homogeneity.

A simple forest plot can be generated by calling the `plot` or `forest.meta` as follows to produce Figure 3.3.

```
> plot(fixed.angina)
```

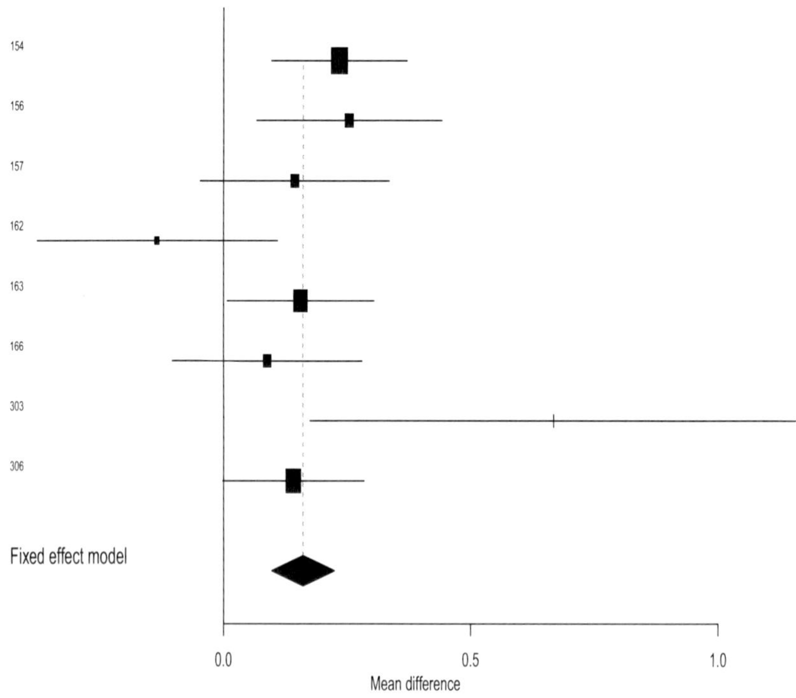

FIGURE 3.3: Default Forest Plot for the Angina Trial with 95% CIs

Figure 3.4 is a better presentation of the forest plot in Figure 3.3, and may be generated by calling `forest.meta` with the R code chunk below.

```
> forest.meta(fixed.angina)
```

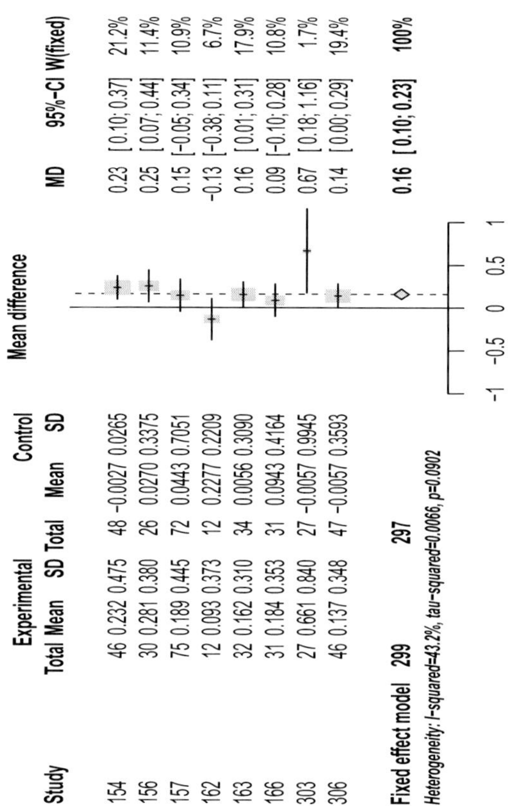

FIGURE 3.4: A Detailed Forest Plot for the Angina Trial with 95% CIs

To assess potential publication bias informally, we generate the funnel plot and visually assess whether it is symmetric. This funnel plot can be generated using the following R code chunk which produces Figure 3.5:

```
> funnel(fixed.angina)
```

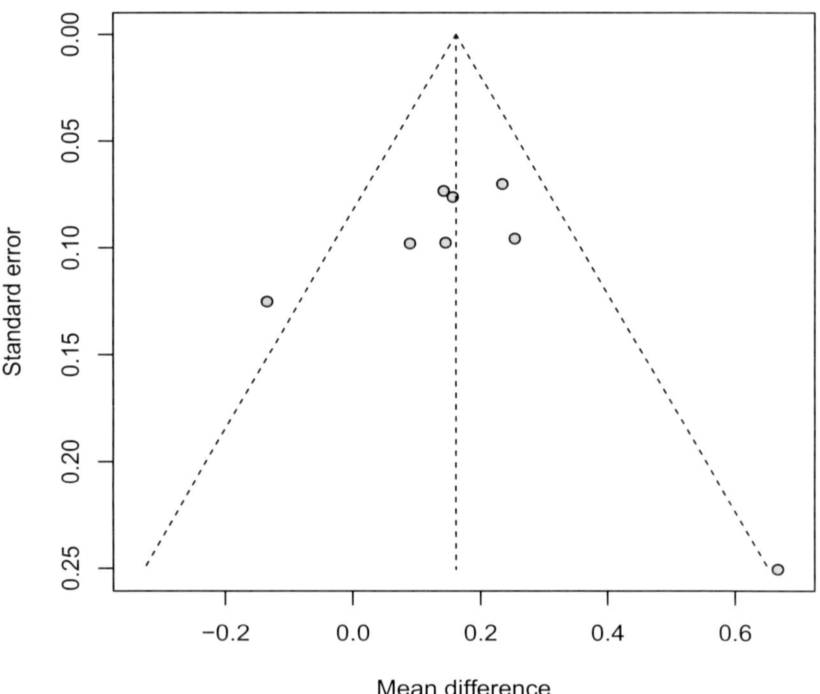

FIGURE 3.5: Funnel Plot for the Angina Trial

From this figure, we note that protocol 303 has the largest mean difference of 0.6669 on the right and protocol 162 has the smallest mean difference of -0.1347 on the left. The remaining are quite symmetric. A statistical significance test can be performed using `metabias`. This test is based on the rank correlation between standardized treatment estimates and variance estimates of estimated treatment effects where Kendall's tau is used as the correlation measure (see from Begg and Mazumdar (1994)). Other tests may be performed and may be seen in the library `meta`.

By calling `metabias` for this model fitting as follows:

```
> metabias(fixed.angina)
```

we see the p-value associated with this test is 0.4579, indicating symmetry of the funnel plot.

3.3.2.3 Fit the Random-Effects Model

Similar to the fixed-effects model in Section 3.3.2.2, we can fit the random-effects model as follows:

```
> # fit random-effects model
> random.angina = metacont(nE, meanE, sqrt(varE),
                           nC,meanC,sqrt(varC),
          data=angina,studlab=Protocol,comb.random=T)
> # print the summary fit
> random.angina
```

```
         MD            95%-CI %W(fixed) %W(random)
154  0.2343  [ 0.0969; 0.372]     21.22      17.47
156  0.2541  [ 0.0663; 0.442]     11.35      12.74
157  0.1451  [-0.0464; 0.337]     10.92      12.45
162 -0.1347  [-0.3798; 0.110]      6.67       9.04
163  0.1566  [ 0.0072; 0.306]     17.94      16.21
166  0.0894  [-0.1028; 0.282]     10.85      12.40
303  0.6669  [ 0.1758; 1.158]      1.66       2.90
306  0.1423  [-0.0015; 0.286]     19.39      16.79

Number of studies combined: k=8
                         MD        95%-CI     z  p.value
Fixed effect model    0.162 [0.0986;0.225] 5.01  <0.0001
Random effects model 0.159 [0.0710;0 247] 3.54   0.0004

Quantifying heterogeneity:
tau^2 = 0.0066; H = 1.33 [1; 2]; I^2 = 43.2% [0%; 74.9%]
```

```
Test of heterogeneity:
     Q d.f.  p.value
 12.33    7   0.0902

Details on meta-analytical method:
- Inverse variance method
- DerSimonian-Laird estimator for tau^2
```

This gives the model fitting for random-effects as well as for fixed-effects. We note from the output that the estimated between-protocol variance $\hat{\tau}^2 = 0.0066$ and that the mean difference is estimated as 0.159 from the random-effects model as compared to 0.162 from the fixed-effects model. The 95% CI from the random-effects model is (0.071, 0.247) as compared to (0.098, 0.225) from the fixed-effects model. Again the 95% CI from the random-effects model is wider than that for the fixed-effects model. We leave generating the forest plot as an exercise for interested readers.

3.4 Which Model Should We Use? Fixed-Effects or Random-Effects?

Whether a fixed-effects model or a random-effects model should be used to synthesize treatment effects across studies in a meta-analysis should not be entirely based upon a test for heterogeneity of treatment effects among the studies. Rather model selection should be based on whether the studies share a common effect size and on the goals in performing the meta-analysis. This requires the analyst to review the studies to be included in the meta-analysis in detail. In fact for the results of a meta-analysis to accrue the highest level of scientific credibility, a protocol (see Chapter 2) should be written to guide all aspects of the meta-analysis as a process: defining the question(s), defining the endpoint(s) or response variable(s), specifying criteria for study inclusion/exclusion, retrieval of study reports, abstracting information from the studies, statistical methods, etc.

3.4.1 Fixed-Effects

In reviewing the studies to be included in a fixed-effects meta-analysis, attention should be given to whether it is reasonable to believe 'a priori' that each study would provide an estimate of the same (or common) treatment effect. If so, then a fixed-effects model may be used.

As an example consider a Phase III, multi-center, randomized, double-blind, controlled clinical trial of a dose of a new drug. Such trials are conducted to confirm efficacy (as compared to control) of the new drug. Patients are randomized to drug or control at each center and all centers follow a common protocol. All patients entered have the same disease and have similar characteristics as defined by the inclusion/exclusion criteria. Although such a trial is usually analyzed using a linear model blocking on center, the trial could be analyzed using a meta-analysis model considering each center as a separate study. Since each center (study) is expected to provide an independent estimate of the same or common treatment effect, a fixed-effects meta-analysis model is reasonable.

3.4.2 Random-Effects

If in reviewing the studies to be included in a meta-analysis, it is unreasonable to believe 'a priori' that each study would provide an estimate of the same (or common) treatment effect, then a random-effects model should be used.

As an example, suppose a pharmaceutical company conducts several randomized, controlled clinical trials of the efficacy of a drug at a given dose in different populations; e.g. six trials in the young ($18 \leq$ age <45), middle ($45 \leq$ age < 65) and old ($65 \leq$ age) age groups of either sex (male, female). It is reasonable to expect that efficacy of the drug will differ across these six populations. Thus a random-effects model would be appropriate to synthesize the estimates of the treatment effect (drug versus control) across the six populations. Note that separate meta-analyses using a random-effects model across age groups could be conducted to obtain the estimate of treatment effect by sex.

3.4.3 Performing Both Fixed-Effects and Random-Effects Meta-Analysis

In practice, many analysts perform both a fixed-effects and a random-effects meta-analysis of the same set of studies - even if there is an 'a priori' basis for believing the fixed-effects model is appropriate. If inference is provided via a confidence interval, generally the confidence interval from the random-effects model analysis will be wider (providing a more conservative inference) than the one from the fixed-effects model analysis. The confidence intervals would be identical only in the case when the inter-study variability (the extent of heterogeneity) is 0. The textbook by Borenstein et al. (2009) as well as The Cochrane Collaborative (`http://www.cochrane-net.org/openlearning/HTML/mod13-4.htm`) and the presentation by Michael Brannick (`http://luna.cas.usf.edu/~mbrannic/files/meta/FixedvRandom.doc`) provide excellent discussion contrasting the fixed-effects versus random-effects cases.

3.5 Summary and Conclusions

In this chapter, we introduced meta-analysis methods for synthesizing studies using publicly available datasets with both fixed-effects and random-effects models. Woolf's test was used to test for lack of homogeneity. Note that this chapter was expanded from chapter 8 in Chen and Peace (2010) with greater detail and better presentation.

Readers of this chapter may use the models and associated R code contained herein to perform their own meta-analyses of studies by synthesizing treatment effects across studies. For further reading, we recommend Hedges and Olkin (1985), Whitehead (2003), Hartung et al. (2008) and Borenstein et al. (2009). For R application, we recommend the reader become more familiar with the `rmeta` and `meta` libraries. There are other R libraries, such as `metacor` for meta-analysis of correlation coefficients and another library of `metafor` for meta-analysis. Chapter 12 (Meta-Analysis) in Everitt and Hothorn (2006) is again an excellent reference on the subject. The commercial software of `Comprehensive Meta-Analysis` associated with the book of Borenstein et al. (2009) is also a must-read in this arena.

Chapter 4

Meta-Analysis with Binary Data

With the conceptual introduction in Chapter 3, we now come to more detailed discussion on meta-analysis for a specific data type. The first and probably most commonly seen meta-analysis is of binary or binomial data where the number of successes are considered in a sequence of independent studies each of which has success with probability p. We begin this chapter with two real datasets in Section 4.1 and then describe the meta-analysis models associated with this type of data in Section 4.2 with step-by-step R implementation using the first dataset. The second dataset will be used in Section 4.3 to illustrate the application of R package `meta` corresponding to the meta-analysis methods detailed in Section 4.2 with discussion in Section 4.4.

Note to the readers: you need to install R packages `gdata` to read in the Excel data file and `meta` for meta-analysis.

4.1 Data from Real Life Studies

4.1.1 Statin Clinical Trials

This study is about meta-analysis of cardiovascular clinical trials designed to compare intensive statin therapy to moderate statin therapy in the reduction of cardiovascular outcomes. The data is from Cannon et al. (2006). Recent clinical trials have demonstrated that high-dose statins (also referred to as intensive statin therapy) appear to be more effective than standard-dose statins in reducing cardiovascular events, as seen in (1) the PROVE IT-TIMI-22 (Pravastatin or Atorvastatin Evaluation and Infection Therapy-Thrombolysis In Myocardial Infarction-22) and (2) the TNT (Treating to

New Targets) trials. However, two trials, (3) the A-to-Z (Aggrastat to Zocor) and (4) the IDEAL (Incremental Decrease in End Points Through Aggressive Lipid Lowering), had non-statistically significant trends toward benefit of intensive statin therapy for their pre-specified primary end point, raising questions regarding the reliability of this observation. In order to determine more accurately the clinical utility of intensive statin therapy, we performed a meta-analysis of these four trials, which represent more than 100,000 patient-years of observation directly comparing high-dose versus standard dose statin therapy. The dataset is shown in Table 4.1.

TABLE 4.1: Data for Coronary Death or MI of Statin Use.

Study	nhigh	evhigh	nstd	evstd	ntot	evtot
Prove It	2099	147	2063	172	4162	319
A-to-Z	2265	205	2232	235	4497	440
TNT	4995	334	5006	418	10001	752
IDEAL	4439	411	4449	463	8888	874

Note that in this table, `nhigh` is the total number of patients randomized to high dose, `evhigh` is the number of patients with event (defined as the combined incidence of coronary death or non-fatal myocardial infarction (MI)) in the high dose group, `nstd` is the total number of patients randomized to standard dose, `evstd` is the number of patients with event in the standard dose group, `ntot` is the total number of patients in both treatment groups, and `evtot` is the total number of patients with events in both treatment groups.

Figure 4.1 summarizes the results of a meta- analysis that shows the relative risk of high dose versus standard dose of statins in preventing death and non-fatal myocardial infarction (MI) from both fixed-effects and random-effects models described in Chapter 3. This analysis is detailed in Section 4.2.1 with the R package `meta`, and we encourage interested readers to read Cannon et al. (2006) which was published in the *Journal of the American College of Cardiology*.

In this figure, the first four rows specify the four individual studies. For

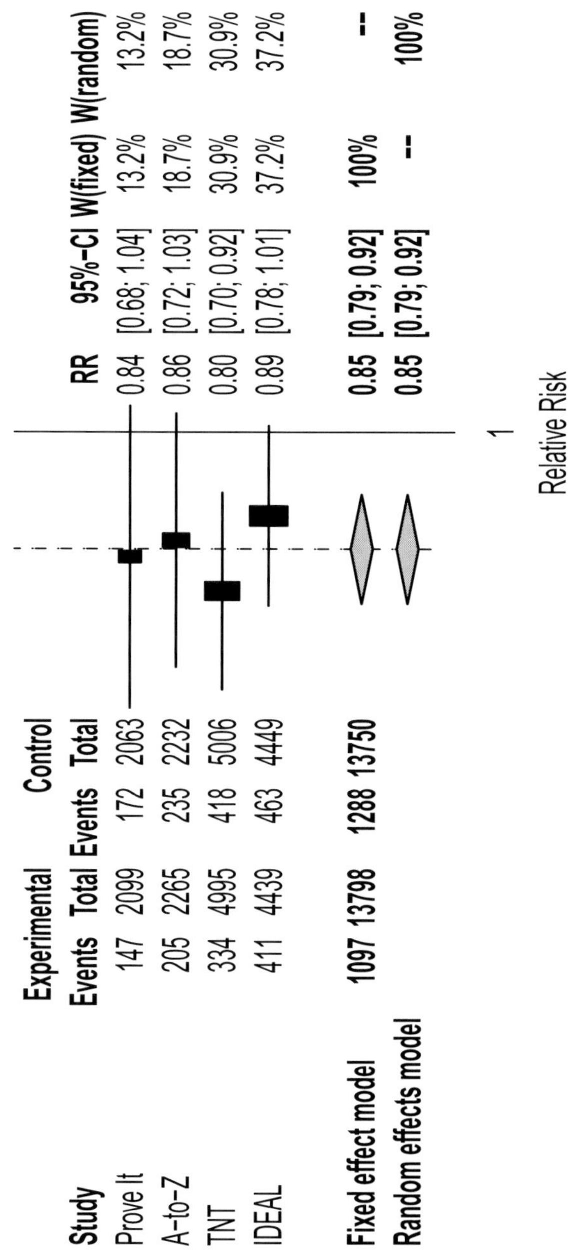

FIGURE 4.1: Meta-Analysis with Risk-Ratio

each, the study name is shown on the left, followed by detailed information of the studies as:

- the observed number of events and total number of patients from both experimental and control groups;
- a forest plot that summarizes all the statistics,
- effect size of relative ratios,
- the 95% confidence intervals,
- the relative weight assigned to the study from both fixed- and random-effect models

Also, the last two rows represent the summary information from both fixed- and random-effects models.

In this chapter, we will use this dataset to illustrate both the detailed steps in implementating the meta-analysis methods and the application of R package `meta` to analyze these data to reproduce the results.

4.1.2 Five Studies on Lamotrigine for Treatment of Bipolar Depression

Bipolar disorder is a psychiatric disorder historically known as manic-depressive disorder. Bipolar disorder is among the top causes of worldwide disability and is characterized by both depressive and manic episodes as described in Geddes et al. (2009). Bipolar disorder is a lifelong recurrent illness and there is no known cure. Patients usually require long-term treatment with psychotherapy drugs to control symptoms. Lamotrigine is one of several drugs used in the treatment of bipolar disorder. It is an anticonvulsant and has been approved by the US FDA as an adjunctive treatment for epilepsy and for maintenance treatment for Bipolar I disorder. Lamotrigine is marketed in the USA and in some European countries as "Lamictal" by GlaxoSmithKline.

Although there is evidence of long-term efficacy of Lamotrigine as maintenance treatment for Bipolar I disorder, five placebo controlled clinical trials of Lamotrigine in acute phase therapy have been reported as individually neutral and there was no statistically significant benefit from this medication as reported in Calabrese et al. (2008). To further investigate the efficacy of lamotrigine in acute bipolar depression, Geddes et al. (2009) conducted a meta-analysis of these five trials (see Table 1 in Geddes) using patient level data. The authors also conducted an extensive database search on MEDLINE, EMBASE, CINAHL, PsyINFO, and CENTRAL and found two more studies which reported substantially statistically significant benefits with lamotrigine. However, these two studies were not used because of substantial differences in protocols. In this chapter, we will illustrate meta-analyses of binary response variables by performing a meta-analysis on two binary response efficacy variables defined in the paper using summary information (count data) from the five placebo controlled trials.

A patient was considered a responder if he/she experienced at least a 50% reduction from baseline in terms of the Hamiliton rating scale for depression (HRSD) or in terms of the Montgomery-Asberg Depression Rating Scale (MADRS). In addition to meta-analyzing these two binary response variables, we also meta-analyze the MADRS response variable according to whether the patient suffered severe depression (HRSD ≥ 24) or mild-to-moderate depression (HRSD < 24) at baseline.

Summary count data on the above four binary response variables from Geddes et al. (2009) were re-typed into the Excel datafile "dat4Meta". The file can be loaded into R as follows:

```
> # Load the library
> require(gdata)
> # Get the excel data book
> datfile = "Your Data Path/dat4Meta.xls"
> # Call "read.xls" to read the specific data
> Lamo  = read.xls(datfile, sheet="Data_Lamo",
                  perl="c:/perl64/bin/perl.exe")
```

The data can be seen from Table 4.2 where `Trial` is the name for the clinical trials, `Events` is the number of patients who responded to "lamotrigine" or "Placebo" as seen in `Group` and `Total` is the total number of patients in the corresponding group. `Response Category` is a variable created to correspond to the four analyses summarized in Figures 1 and 2 of the Geddes et al., where `1` is for $> 50\%$ reduction in Hamilton Rating Scale for Depression (HRSD), `2` for $> 50\%$ reduction on Montgomery-Asberg Depression Rating

TABLE 4.2: Data for Five Lamotrigine Clinical Trials.

Trial	Events	Total	Group	Category
SCA100223	59	111	lamotrigine	1
SCA30924	47	131	lamotrigine	1
SCA40910	51	133	lamotrigine	1
SCAA2010	51	103	lamotrigine	1
SCAB2001	32	63	lamotrigine	1
SCA100223	44	109	placebo	1
SCA30924	37	128	placebo	1
SCA40910	39	124	placebo	1
SCAA2010	45	103	placebo	1
SCAB2001	21	66	placebo	1
SCA100223	59	111	lamotrigine	2
SCA30924	56	131	lamotrigine	2
SCA40910	55	133	lamotrigine	2
SCAA2010	51	103	lamotrigine	2
SCAB2001	31	63	lamotrigine	2
SCA100223	44	109	placebo	2
SCA30924	44	128	placebo	2
SCA40910	47	124	placebo	2
SCAA2010	46	103	placebo	2
SCAB2001	19	66	placebo	2
SCA100223	25	57	lamotrigine	3
SCA30924	32	65	lamotrigine	3
SCA40910	34	86	lamotrigine	3
SCAA2010	31	56	lamotrigine	3
SCAB2001	20	35	lamotrigine	3
SCA100223	29	65	placebo	3
SCA30924	26	62	placebo	3
SCA40910	31	76	placebo	3
SCAA2010	31	60	placebo	3
SCAB2001	14	31	placebo	3
SCA100223	34	54	lamotrigine	4
SCA30924	24	66	lamotrigine	4
SCA40910	21	47	lamotrigine	4
SCAA2010	20	47	lamotrigine	4
SCAB2001	11	28	lamotrigine	4
SCA100223	17	44	placebo	4
SCA30924	18	66	placebo	4
SCA40910	16	48	placebo	4
SCAA2010	15	43	placebo	4
SCAB2001	5	35	placebo	4

Scale (MADRS), 3 for MADRS response for baseline Hamilton Rating Scale for Depression < 24, and 4 for MADRS response for baseline Hamilton Rating Scale for Depression ≥ 24.

This dataset will be used to illustrate meta-analyses using the `R meta` package. We will first reproduce the results from the paper using the risk ratio as the treatment effect, followed by meta-analyses using the risk-difference and odds ratio as treatment effects.

4.2 Meta-Analysis Methods

A goal of meta-analysis is to combine estimates of treatment effect or effect sizes (ESs) across similar studies. If estimates of treatment effect or effect size are not provided, but the number of patients responding out of the total number studied on treatment and control are, we have to calculate the effect size for each study, and then combine the effect sizes to assess the consistency of the effect across studies and to compute a summary effect.

Commonly used ESs for binomial data are the risk ratio, the risk-difference, and the odds ratio. We will discuss these ESs in meta-analyses conducted.

4.2.1 Analysis with Risk-Ratio

4.2.1.1 Definition

The effect size for the risk-ratio (RR) of one treatment (such as "Experimental") to another (such as "Control") is defined as:

$$ES = \frac{p_E}{p_C} = \frac{x_E/n_E}{x_C/n_C} \tag{4.1}$$

where p_E is the so-called risk (or risk probability) for the experimental treatment (E) which is computed as the total number of events (x_E) divided by the total number of patients (n_E), i.e. $p_E = \frac{x_E}{n_E}$ with similar notations for control (C).

Corresponding to the statin data in Section 4.1.1, a risk-ratio of 1 means that the risk of death or MI was the same in both groups, while a risk- ratio less than 1.0 would mean that the risk was lower in the high-dose group, and a risk-ratio greater than 1.0 would mean that the risk was lower in the standard-dose group.

To construct an approximate confidence interval based on the normal distribution, ES is transformed using the natural logarithm and then employing the delta-method where $lnES = ln(ES)$. The variance for $lnES$ can be shown to be

$$Var_{lnES} = \frac{1}{x_E} - \frac{1}{n_E} + \frac{1}{x_C} - \frac{1}{n_C} \tag{4.2}$$

This is accomplished by representing $lnES$ as the linear terms in a Taylor series expansion about its expected value as:

$$\begin{aligned}
lnES &= lnES(x_E, x_C) = ln(p_E) - ln(p_C) \\
&= ln(x_E) - ln(n_E) - ln(x_C) + ln(n_C) \\
&= lnES(\mu_{x_E}, \mu_{x_C}) + \left(\frac{\partial lnES}{\partial x_E}\right)_{\mu_E} (x_E - \mu_{x_E}) \\
&\quad + \left(\frac{\partial lnES}{\partial x_C}\right)_{\mu_C} (x_C - \mu_{x_C})
\end{aligned}$$

Then

$$\begin{aligned}
Var(lnES) &= \left(\frac{\partial lnES}{\partial x_E}\right)^2_{\mu_E} Var(x_E) + \left(\frac{\partial lnES}{\partial x_C}\right)^2_{\mu_C} Var(x_C) \\
&= \left(\frac{1}{n_E p_E}\right)^2 n_E p_E (1 - p_E) + \left(\frac{1}{n_C p_C}\right)^2 n_C p_C (1 - p_C) \\
&= \frac{1}{n_E p_E}(1 - p_E) + \frac{1}{n_C p_C}(1 - p_C) \\
&= \frac{1}{n_E p_E}(1 - p_E) - \frac{1}{n_E} + \frac{1}{n_C p_C}(1 - p_C) - \frac{1}{n_C}
\end{aligned}$$

which is simplified to be equation (4.2). Therefore, the approximated standard error is

$$SE_{lnES} = \sqrt{Var(lnES)} \tag{4.3}$$

With this, the 95% CI for $lnES$ can be expressed as

$$(lnES - 1.96 \times SE_{lnES}, lnES + 1.96 \times SE_{lnES}). \tag{4.4}$$

We then transform back to the original scale for risk- ratio(RR) as:

$$RR = exp(lnES)$$
$$L_{RR} = exp(lnES - 1.96 \times SE_{lnES})$$
$$U_{RR} = exp(lnES + 1.96 \times SE_{lnES})$$

For illustration with this data, the risks for experimental high-dose group are:

```
> # The events
> xE = dat$evhigh
> # the total number
> nE = dat$nhigh
> # the risk
> pE = xE/nE
> # print the risk
> pE

[1] 0.0700 0.0905 0.0669 0.0926
```

And the risks from the standard low-dose group are:

```
> xC = dat$evstd
> nC = dat$nstd
> pC = xC/nC
> pC

[1] 0.0834 0.1053 0.0835 0.1041
```

And we can see generally that the risk for the experimental high-dose group is lower than the standard low-dose group. Then the risk-ratios are calculated as:

```
> # The risk-ratios
> ES = pE/pC
> # print the RR
> ES

[1] 0.840 0.860 0.801 0.890
```

Again the ratios are smaller than 1 for all four studies indicating the experimental treatment is descriptively better than the standard treatment.

4.2.1.2 Statistical Significance

With the definition and calculations above, we can assess whether the ESs are statistically significant or not. We have several ways to do this.

1. **Confidence Interval Approach**

   The first way is to use a confidence interval. The confidence interval is usually started with the log risk-ratio to use the normal approximation. The log-ES and its variance can be calculated using R as follows:

```
> # calculate the log risk-ratio
> lnES = log(ES)
> # print the log risk-ratio
> lnES

[1] -0.174 -0.151 -0.222 -0.117

> # calculate the variance
> VlnES = 1/dat$evhigh - 1/dat$nhigh + 1/dat$evstd - 1/dat$nstd
> # print the variance
> VlnES

[1] 0.01166 0.00824 0.00499 0.00414
```

   With these calculations, we can construct the 95% CI for $lnES$ as follows:

```
> # upper CI
> ciup  = lnES+1.96*sqrt(VlnES)
> print(ciup)

[1]  0.03724  0.02671 -0.08374  0.00927

> # lower CI
> cilow  = lnES-1.96*sqrt(VlnES)
> print(cilow)

[1] -0.386 -0.329 -0.361 -0.243
```

```
> # then transform back to the original scale
> cat("The low CI is:", exp(cilow),"\n\n")

The low CI is: 0.68 0.719 0.697 0.784

> cat("The upper CI is:", exp(ciup),"\n\n")

The upper CI is: 1.04 1.03 0.92 1.01
```

We can see from the 95% CI that only the study *TNT* (i.e. the third study) is statistically significant and the other three are not. Corresponding to the Figure 4.1, the effect size for each study is represented by a square, with the location of the square representing both the direction and magnitude of the effect. Here, the effect size for each study falls to the left of the center line (indicating a benefit for the high-dose group). The effect is strongest (most distant from the center) in the *TNT* study and weakest in the *IDEAL* study.

2. **The p-value Approach**

   The second way is to calculate the classical p-values. To calculate the p-values, we first calculate the z-values as follows:

```
> # The z-value
> z = lnES/sqrt(VlnES)
> # Print the z-values
> z

[1] -1.62 -1.67 -3.15 -1.82
```

Then the p-values can be calculated as:

```
> pval = 2*(1-pnorm(abs(z)))
> cat("p-values = ", pval, sep=" ", "\n\n")

p-values =  0.106 0.0957 0.00166 0.0694
```

Again, only the study *TNT* is statistically significant at the 5% level.

3. **The Post-Power Approach**

   Looking into the data, we can easily see that the sample sizes for *TNT*, *IDEAL*, *Prove It* and *A-to-Z* are 10,001, 8,888, 4,162 and 4,497, respectively. The *TNT* has the largest sample size which would have greater power to detect statistically significant effect. We can calculate a statistical post- power for these four studies using the R package `pwr` as follows:

```
> # load the pwr library
> library(pwr)
> # calculate the power and print it
> pow.study = pwr.2p2n.test(ES.h(pE,pC),n1=dat$nhigh,
         n2=dat$nstd,sig.level=0.05)
> pow.study

     difference of proportion power calculation for
         binomial distribution (arcsine transformation)
              h = 0.0502, 0.0498, 0.0632, 0.0386
             n1 = 2099, 2265, 4995, 4439
             n2 = 2063, 2232, 5006, 4449
      sig.level = 0.05
          power = 0.367, 0.386, 0.885, 0.444
    alternative = two.sided
 NOTE: different sample sizes
```

   We can see that the associated statistical power for Study *TNT* is 0.885 and the rest of the three studies are all about 40%, indicating these studies are low-powered statistically.

4.2.1.3 The Risk-Ratio Meta-Analysis: Step-by-Step

To increase precision and statistical power to detect a statistically significant effect size, we conduct a meta- analysis of the effect sizes across the individual studies. We first review some relevant concepts used in both fixed-effects and random-effects meta-analysis models and show step-by-step calculations in R.

The precision in meta-analysis can be addressed in two ways with one as the confidence interval and another as the standard error of the ES. Both are in fact related. As depicted in Figure 4.1, the effect size for each study is bounded by a confidence interval, reflecting the precision with which the effect size has been estimated in that study. The confidence interval for the last study (*IDEAL*) is noticeably narrower than that for the first study (*Prove-It*), reflecting the fact that the Ideal study has greater precision. Another way is to observe the size of the variances or standard errors. For these studies, the variance for the log risk ratio of $lnES$ are:

```
> VlnES

[1] 0.01166 0.00824 0.00499 0.00414
```

Again, we can see the last two studies have the smallest variances indicating greater precision. Studies with greater precision should have larger weights when combining studies. This may be done by using a fixed-effects meta-analysis model and weighting each study by its inverse variance as:

$$w_i = \frac{1}{Var_i} \tag{4.5}$$

where $i = 1, \cdots, K = 4$. For these studies, the inverse weights are calculated as:

```
> # Inverse weighting
> w = 1/VlnES
> w

[1]  85.8 121.3 200.5 241.4
```

In Figure 4.1, the solid squares that are used to depict each of the studies vary in size, reflecting the weight that is assigned to the corresponding study in computing the summary effect. The *TNT* and *IDEAL* studies are assigned relatively large weights, while a somewhat lower weight is assigned to the *A to Z* study and less still to the *Prove-It* study.

As one would expect, there is a relationship between a study's precision and that study's weight in the combined analysis. Studies with relatively good precision (*TNT* and *IDEAL*) are assigned greater weights while studies with relatively poor precision (*Prove-It*) are assigned lesser weights. Since precision is driven primarily by sample size, we can think of the studies as being weighted by sample size, where the last two studies have the larger weights.

The fixed-effects weighted average meta-analysis model to combine the studies is then derived as:

$$lnES = \frac{\sum_{i=1}^{4} lnES_i \times w_i}{\sum_{i=1}^{4} w_i} \tag{4.6}$$

with variance calculated by:

$$Var(lnES) = \frac{1}{\sum_{i=1}^{4} w_i} \tag{4.7}$$

The calculations can be performed step by step as follows:

```
> # the inverse of variance for each study
> fwi = 1/VlnES
> fwi

[1]  85.8 121.3 200.5 241.4

> # the total weight
> fw = sum(fwi)
> fw

[1] 649

> # the relative weight for each study
> rw = fwi/fw
> rw

[1] 0.132 0.187 0.309 0.372

> # the weighted mean
> flnES = sum(lnES*rw)
> flnES

[1] -0.163

> # the variance for the weighted mean
> var= 1/fw;
> var
```

```
[1] 0.00154
```

We then transform back to the original scale to estimate the RR as well as the CI as:

```
> # the RR
> exp(flnES)

[1] 0.849

> # the lower and upper CI bounds
> exp(flnES-1.96*sqrt(var))
[1] 0.786
> exp(flnES+1.96*sqrt(var))
[1] 0.917
```

This CI is below the RR of 1 which indicates that the high- dose regimen is statistically significantly more effective than the standard dose regimen.

To illustrate the random-effects meta-model, we first need to estimate the heterogeneity statistic Q in equation (3.18) as:

```
> # estimate heterogeneity statistic Q
> Q = sum(fwi*lnES^2)-(sum(fwi*lnES))^2/fw
> Q

[1] 1.24

> # Get the degrees of freedom
> K  = dim(dat)[1]; df = K -1
> df

[1] 3

> # calculate the statistical significance: p-value
> pval4Q =  pchisq(Q, df, lower.tail=F)
> pval4Q

[1] 0.743
```

From this p-value, we can conclude that there is no statistically significant heterogeneity among these 4 studies. Furthermore since this estimated Q is less than the df of 3, the estimated τ^2 in equation (3.18) is then set to zero which would lead to the conclusion that the random-effects meta-analysis is exactly the same as the fixed-effects model.

4.2.1.4 Risk-Ratio Meta-Analysis: R package `meta`

All the above calculations can be summarized in the R package `meta` in this one-line code where `Inverse` weighting `method` is used for "summary method" `sm="RR"`:

```
> # call "metabin" for RR meta-analysis
> RR.Statin = metabin(evhigh,nhigh,evstd,nstd,studlab=Study,
  data=dat, method="Inverse", sm="RR")
> # print the analysis summary
> summary(RR.Statin)

Number of studies combined: k=4
                         RR           95%-CI     z  p.value
Fixed effect model    0.849   [0.786; 0.917] -4.16 < 0.0001
Random effects model 0.849   [0.786; 0.917] -4.16 < 0.0001


Quantifying heterogeneity:
tau^2 < 0.0001; H = 1 [1; 1.64]; I^2 = 0% [0%; 63%]
Test of heterogeneity:
    Q d.f.  p.value
 1.24    3   0.7428
Details on meta-analytical method:
- Inverse variance method
- DerSimonian-Laird estimator for tau^2
```

Readers can check the results from this output with the step- by-step calculations in Section 4.2.1.3 and should find the results to match exactly.

The forest plot in Figure 4.1 is then produced as follows:

```
> forest(RR.Statin)
```

4.2.2 Analysis with Risk-Difference

4.2.2.1 Definition

Even though the risk-ratio is the most commonly used in binomial data, the risk difference is an ES which is easily understandable. The definition of risk difference (RD) is simply the difference of the risks between two treatments as:

$$ES_{RD} = \hat{p}_E - \hat{p}_C = \frac{x_E}{n_E} - \frac{x_C}{n_C} \tag{4.8}$$

from the notations from previous section.

The variance of ES_{RD} can be estimated as:

$$Var\left(ES_{RD}\right) = \frac{\hat{p}_E(1-\hat{p}_E)}{n_E} + \frac{\hat{p}_C(1-\hat{p}_C)}{n_C} \tag{4.9}$$

and the standard error (SE) is then calculated as $SE_{ES_{RD}} = \sqrt{Var\left(ES_{RD}\right)}$. With the point estimate from equation (4.8) and its variance in equation (4.9), we can frame the same procedures for statistical inference similar to those in Section 4.2.1.2.

For the statin data in Section 4.1.1, a risk difference of 0 means that the risk of death or MI was the same in both groups, while a risk ratio less than 0 means that the risk was lower in the high-dose group, and a risk ratio greater than 0 means that the risk was lower in the standard-dose group. The risk difference can be calculated as:

```
> # the risk difference
> ESRD = pE-pC
> ESRD

[1] -0.0133 -0.0148 -0.0166 -0.0115
```

The differences are less than 0 for all four studies indicating that the experimental treatment is descriptively better than the standard treatment. The variance can be calculated as:

```
> # calculate the variance
> VarRD = pE*(1-pE)/nE + pC*(1-pC)/nC
> VarRD

[1] 6.81e-05 7.85e-05 2.78e-05 3.99e-05
```

```
> # calculate the standard error
> SERD = sqrt(VarRD)
> SERD

[1] 0.00825 0.00886 0.00527 0.00632
```

The step-by-step calculations for RD are left to interested readers. We now illustrate use of the R package `meta`.

4.2.2.2 Implementation in R Package `meta`

The same R function `metabin` is called with `sm` (i.e. "summary method") now set to `RD`:

```
> # call metabin for RD meta-analysis
> RD.Statin = metabin(evhigh,nhigh,evstd,nstd,studlab=Study,
  data=dat, method="Inverse", sm="RD")
> # print the summary
> summary(RD.Statin)

Number of studies combined: k=4
                          RD          95%-CI      z  p.value
Fixed effect model    -0.014 [-0.021;-0.008] -4.27 < 0.0001
Random effects model -0.014 [-0.021;-0.008] -4.27 < 0.0001
Quantifying heterogeneity:
tau^2 < 0.0001; H = 1 [1; 1]; I^2 = 0% [0%; 0%]
Test of heterogeneity:
    Q d.f.  p.value
 0.41    3   0.9379
Details on meta-analytical method:
- Inverse variance method
- DerSimonian-Laird estimator for tau^2
```

The conclusions from the meta-analysis of the risk ratio (RR) are reached from the meta-analysis of the risk difference (RD); i.e. the high-dose regimen is statistically more effective than the standard dose regimen. With this RD meta- analysis, the forest plot can be shown in Figure 4.2 as follows:

```
> forest(RD.Statin)
```

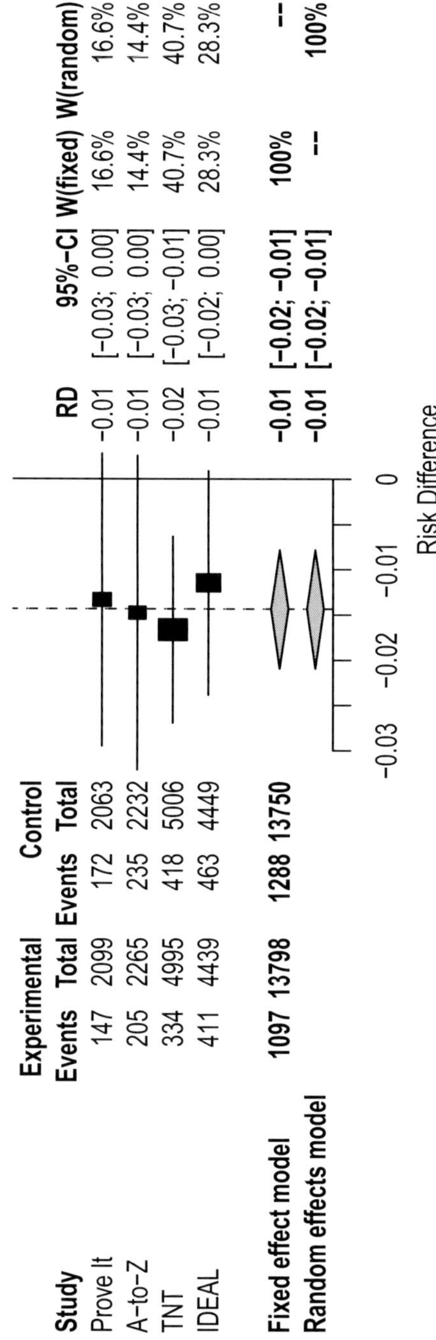

FIGURE 4.2: Meta-Analysis with Risk Difference

4.2.3 Meta-Analysis with Odds Ratio

4.2.3.1 Data Structure

The definition of odds ratio starts with a 2 by 2 table which is usually used to report the number of events and non-events in two groups.

From a total of K studies, the data from the ith study ($i = 1, \cdots, K$) can be represented as cells A_i, B_i, C_i, and D_i, as shown in Table 4.3.

TABLE 4.3: Nomenclature for 2×2 Table of Outcome by Treatment.

	Events	Non-Events	Total Event
Experimental (High Dose)	A_i	B_i	n_1
Standard (Low Dose)	C_i	D_i	n_2

For example, the data from the TNT study can be seen in Table 4.4.

TABLE 4.4: Data from TNT.

	MI	No-MI	Total
High Dose	334	4995-334	4995
Low Dose	418	5006-418	5006

4.2.3.2 Odds Ratio: Woolf's Method

The odds ratio (OR) associated with an event is defined as the ratio of the odds of the event in one study group to the odds of the event in another study group. The odds of the event for the treatment group in the ith study is

$$OddsE_i = \frac{p_{E_i}}{1-p_{E_i}} = \frac{\frac{A_i}{A_i+B_i}}{1-\frac{A_i}{A_i+B_i}} = \frac{\frac{A_i}{A_i+B_i}}{\frac{B_i}{A_i+B_i}} = \frac{A_i}{B_i} \tag{4.10}$$

Similarly the odds of the event for the control group in the ith study is

$$OddsC_i = \frac{p_{C_i}}{1-p_{C_i}} = \frac{\frac{C_i}{C_i+D_i}}{1-\frac{C_i}{C_i+D_i}} = \frac{\frac{C_i}{C_i+D_i}}{\frac{D_i}{C_i+D_i}} = \frac{C_i}{D_i} \tag{4.11}$$

Then the odds ratio (OR) of the treatment group to the control group for ith study is as follows:

$$OR_i = \frac{OddsE_i}{OddsC_i} = \frac{\frac{A_i}{B_i}}{\frac{C_i}{D_i}} = \frac{A_iD_i}{B_iC_i} \tag{4.12}$$

For the statin studies, the odds of MI in the experimental high-dose group is

```
> oddsE = pE/(1-pE)
> oddsE

[1] 0.0753 0.0995 0.0717 0.1020
```

and the odds of MI in the standard low-dose group is

```
> oddsC = pC/(1-pC)
> oddsC

[1] 0.0910 0.1177 0.0911 0.1162
```

The OR would then be

```
> OR = oddsE/oddsC
> OR

[1] 0.828 0.846 0.787 0.878
```

Readers may find the odds ratio intuitively less appealing than the RR or RD. However the odds ratio is used in many statistically sound analysis methods, especially in logistic regression. It is commonly used as a measure of effect size in analyzing categorical data in the form of 2 by 2 tables including the meta-analyses of binomial data in this chapter. For the case when the risk of the event is low, the odds ratio is close to the risk ratio.

To approximate the normal distribution in using odds ratios, we usually convert the odds ratio to the log scale and estimate the log odds ratio and its standard error and use these numbers to perform the meta-analysis. Then we transform the results back into the original metric.

With this direction, the log odds ratio is

$$LogOR = ln(OR) \tag{4.13}$$

The approximate variance can be derived from delta method from the definition as follows:

$$OR = \frac{AD}{BC} = \frac{\frac{\hat{P}_E}{1-\hat{P}_E}}{\frac{\hat{P}_C}{1-\hat{P}_C}} \tag{4.14}$$

and the log odds ratio is

$$\begin{aligned} logOR &= ln(OR) = ln\left(\frac{\hat{P}_E}{1-\hat{P}_E}\right) - ln\left(\frac{\hat{P}_C}{1-\hat{P}_C}\right) \\ &= f(\hat{P}_E) - f(\hat{P}_C) \end{aligned} \tag{4.15}$$

where $f(x) = ln\left(\frac{x}{1-x}\right)$ with derivative as $f'(x) = -\frac{1}{x(1-x)}$

The approximate variance can be derived using the delta method to expand (via Taylor series) the log-odds for both treatment and control about their expected values as

$$\begin{aligned} logOR &= ln\left(\frac{\hat{P}_E}{1-\hat{P}_E}\right) - ln\left(\frac{\hat{P}_C}{1-\hat{P}_C}\right) \\ &\approx \left[f(P_E) + f'(P_E)(\hat{P}_E - P_E)\right] - \left[f(P_C) + f'(P_C)(\hat{P}_C - P_C)\right] \\ &= \left[f(P_E) - \frac{1}{P_E(1-P_E)}(\hat{P}_E - P_E)\right] \\ &\quad - \left[f(P_C) - \frac{1}{P_C(1-P_C)}(\hat{P}_C - P_C)\right] \end{aligned} \tag{4.16}$$

The variance can then be obtained as follows:

$$\begin{aligned} var(logOR) &= \left[\frac{1}{P_E(1-P_E)}\right]^2 var(\hat{P}_E - P_E) \\ &\quad + \left[\frac{1}{P_C(1-P_C)}\right]^2 var(\hat{P}_C - P_C) \\ &= \left[\frac{1}{P_E(1-P_E)}\right]^2 \frac{P_E(1-P_E)}{n_E} \\ &\quad + \left[\frac{1}{P_C(1-P_C)}\right]^2 \frac{P_C(1-P_C)}{n_C} \\ &= \frac{1}{n_E P_E(1-P_E)} + \frac{1}{n_C P_C(1-P_C)} \\ &= \frac{1}{n_E \frac{A}{n_E}\frac{B}{n_E}} + \frac{1}{n_C \frac{C}{n_C}\frac{D}{n_C}} \\ &= \frac{n_T}{AB} + \frac{n_C}{CD} = \frac{1}{A} + \frac{1}{B} + \frac{1}{C} + \frac{1}{D} \end{aligned} \tag{4.17}$$

Therefore the approximate standard error is:

$$SE_{logOR} = \sqrt{V_{logOR}} \tag{4.18}$$

With these calculations in the log-scale, we then transform them back to original scale for odds ratios (OR) using

$$OR = exp(logOR) \tag{4.19}$$

$$LL_{OR} = exp(LL_{logOR}) \tag{4.20}$$

and

$$UL_{OR} = exp(LL_{logOR}) \tag{4.21}$$

where LL and UL represent the lower and upper limits, respectively.

Now we illustrate the calculations using the TNT study. For this study, the OR for the 4 studies are

```
> OR
```

```
[1] 0.828 0.846 0.787 0.878
```

and then the log odds ratios are

```
> LogOR= log(OR)
> LogOR
```

```
[1] -0.189 -0.168 -0.240 -0.130
```

The approximate variance can be calculated as $V_{LogOR} = \frac{1}{334} + \frac{1}{4995-334} + \frac{1}{418} + \frac{1}{5006-418}$ as:

```
> VLogOR = 1/334+ 1/(4995-334)+1/418+1/(5006-418)
> VLogOR
```

```
[1] 0.00582
```

and standard error

```
> SE.LogOR=sqrt(VLogOR)
> SE.LogOR
```

```
[1] 0.0763
```

The weightings from both fixed-effects and random-effects models can be easily implemented. We leave these as exercises for interested readers. We will now use the R package `meta` for meta-analysis of OR.

4.2.3.3 R Implementation with R Package meta

The OR meta-analysis can be easily implemented in this package with the following code where `sm="OR"` is used to call "OR":

```
> OR.Statin = metabin(evhigh,nhigh,evstd,nstd,studlab=Study,
  data=dat, method="Inverse", sm="OR")
> summary(OR.Statin)

Number of studies combined: k=4


                         OR           95%-CI     z  p.value
Fixed effect model    0.835  [0.768; 0.909] -4.18 < 0.0001
Random effects model 0.835  [0.768; 0.909] -4.18 < 0.0001

Quantifying heterogeneity:
tau^2 < 0.0001; H = 1 [1; 1.58]; I^2 = 0% [0%; 59.7%]

Test of heterogeneity:
    Q d.f.  p.value
 1.14    3   0.7673

Details on meta-analytical method:
- Inverse variance method
- DerSimonian-Laird estimator for tau^2
```

The forest plot can be shown as in Figure 4.3 as follows:

```
> forest(OR.Statin)
```

4.2.4 Meta-Analysis using Mantel-Haenszel Method

4.2.4.1 Details of the Mantel-Haenszel Method

As an alternative, the Mantel-Haenszel(MH) method may be used to provide an estimate of the pooled odds ratio across the studies (summarized as 2 by 2 tables) under a fixed-effects model. The MH pooled odds ratio is defined

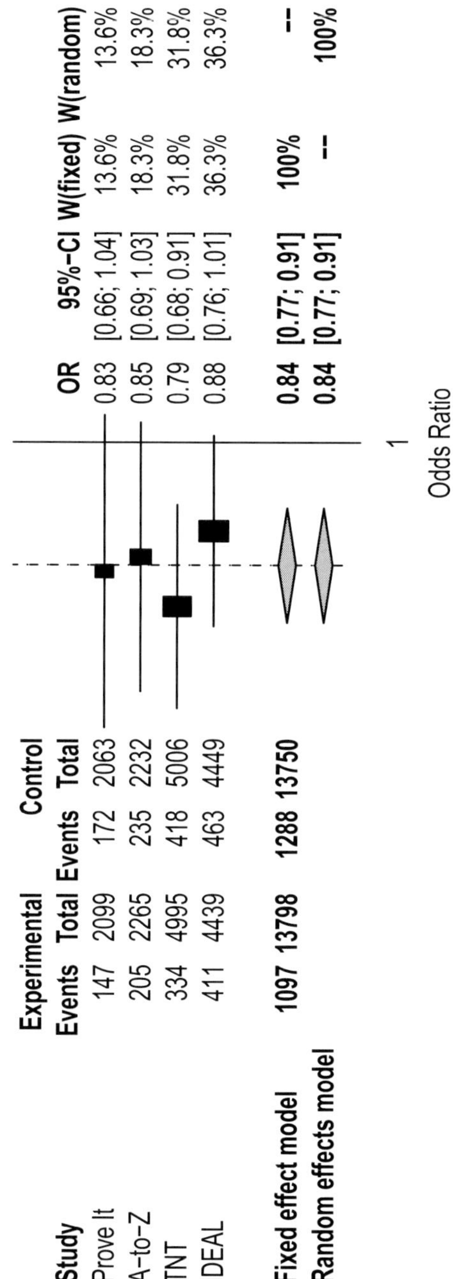

FIGURE 4.3: Meta-Analysis with Odds Ratio with Inverse-Weighting

as follows:

$$\widehat{OR}_{MH} = \frac{\sum_{i=1}^{K}\left(\frac{A_iD_i}{N_i}\right)}{\sum_{i=1}^{K}\left(\frac{B_iC_i}{N_i}\right)} \tag{4.22}$$

where $N_i = A_i + B_i + C_i + D_i$

There are alternative fixed-effects methods, such as Woolf and inverse variance. However, the Mantel-Haenszel method is generally regarded as more robust, particularly when cell counts are small and the number of studies is large.

The pooled MH odds ratio defined above is in fact a weighted average of the odds ratios from the individual studies. This can be seen from re-arranging the MH equation (4.22) and using the equation (4.12) as follows:

$$\begin{aligned}
\widehat{OR}_{MH} &= \frac{\sum_{i=1}^{K}\left(\frac{B_iC_i}{N_i}\frac{A_iD_i}{B_iC_i}\right)}{\sum_{i=1}^{K}\left(\frac{B_iC_i}{N_i}\right)} = \frac{\sum_{i=1}^{K}\left(\frac{B_iC_i}{N_i} \times OR_i\right)}{\sum_{i=1}^{K}\left(\frac{B_iC_i}{N_i}\right)} \\
&= \sum_{i=1}^{K}\left(\frac{\frac{B_iC_i}{N_i}}{\sum_{i=1}^{K}\left(\frac{B_iC_i}{N_i}\right)}\right) \times OR_i \\
&= \sum_{i=1}^{K} relWeight_i \times OR_i
\end{aligned} \tag{4.23}$$

where the weight is defined as $wt_i = \frac{B_iC_i}{N_i}$ and the relative weight is defined as $relWeight_i = \frac{\frac{B_iC_i}{N_i}}{\sum_{i=1}^{K}\left(\frac{B_iC_i}{N_i}\right)}$ with total weight as $totalWeight = \frac{1}{\sum_{i=1}^{K}\left(\frac{B_iC_i}{N_i}\right)}$.

Note that the weight of $wt_i = \frac{B_iC_i}{N_i}$ is the inverse of the variance of OR_i for each study when the $OR = 1$, which is to say that the weight is related to the variance in a special form when there is no association. Because Mantel-Haenszel works well in many applications and is much simpler, it is often favored in the statistical analysis of binomial data.

Recall from the derivation of inverse-weighting, this total weight is in fact the variance of MH estimator as

$$Var\left(\widehat{OR}_{MH}\right) = totalWeight = \frac{1}{\sum_{i=1}^{K}\left(\frac{B_iC_i}{N_i}\right)} \tag{4.24}$$

Therefore, the 95% confidence interval for the Mantel- Haenszel odds ratio may be calculated as:

$$\widehat{OR}_{MH} \pm 1.96\sqrt{Var\left(\widehat{OR}_{MH}\right)} \tag{4.25}$$

Although the MH OR estimate has many advantages and statistical properties, it is used to estimate the odds ratio instead of log odds ratio. Its distribution is not symmetric and the normal distribution is not appropriate for constructing confidence intervals. Emerson (1994) proposed to use the variance estimate from Robins et al. (1986) for the log odds ratio to provide a confidence interval for this meta odds ratio. Denote the $\hat{\theta}$ as the estimated log odds ratio where $\hat{\theta} = log(OR)$, then the variance estimate can be obtained as:

$$Var(\hat{\theta}) = \frac{1}{2}\sum_{i=1}^{K}\left(\frac{T_{1i}T_{3i}}{ST_3^2} + \frac{T_{1i}T_{4i} + T_{2i}T_{3i}}{ST_3ST_4} + \frac{T_{2i}T_{4i}}{ST_4^2}\right) \tag{4.26}$$

where $T_{1i} = \frac{A_i+D_i}{N_i}$, $T_{2i} = \frac{B_i+C_i}{N_i}$, $T_{3i} = \frac{A_iD_i}{N_i}$, $T_{4i} = \frac{B_iC_i}{N_i}$, $ST_3 = \sum_{i=1}^{K} T_{3i}$ and $ST_4 = \sum_{i=1}^{K} T_{4i}$.

4.2.4.2 Step-by-Step R Implementation

We have obtained the odds ratios from previous section as:

```
> OR

[1] 0.828 0.846 0.787 0.878
```

To calculate the relative weighting from each study, we first calculate $\frac{B_iC_i}{N_i}$ as:

```
> w0 = (dat$nhigh-dat$evhigh)*dat$evstd/(dat$nhigh+dat$nstd)
> w0

[1]  80.7 107.6 194.8 209.8
```

The total weights can then be calculated as:

```
> TotWeight = sum(w0)
> TotWeight

[1] 593
```

With this total weight, we can compute the relative weighting as:

```
> relWt = w0/TotWeight
> relWt
```

```
[1] 0.136 0.182 0.329 0.354
```

The MH OR estimate across the studies is then calculated as:

```
> OR.MH = sum(relWt*OR)
> OR.MH

[1] 0.835
```

We will demonstrate both the naive and the Emerson approaches to calculate the variance.

As the naive approach to use the inverse of the total weight as the variance, the variance is:

```
> Var.ORMH1 = 1/TotWeight
> Var.ORMH1

[1] 0.00169
```

Therefore the 95% CI can be computed as:

```
> lowCI = OR.MH-1.96*sqrt(Var.ORMH1)
> upCI = OR.MH+1.96*sqrt(Var.ORMH1)

> cat("MH estimate=", round(OR.MH,4),sep="", "\n\n")

MH estimate=0.835

> cat("The 95% CI for MH =(", round(lowCI, 4), ",",
 round(upCI, 4), ")", sep="", "\n\n")

The 95% CI for MH =(0.755,0.916)
```

Since this approximation is not good as discussed, we will use Emerson's approximation. Let's first get the data:

```
> A = dat$evhigh;  B  = dat$nhigh-dat$evhigh
> C = dat$evstd;   D = dat$nstd - dat$evstd
> N = A+B+C+D
```

And then calculate the quantities from the Emerson approximation as follows:

```
> T1 = (A+D)/N;  T2 = (B+C)/N
> T3 = A*D/N;    T4 = B*C/N
> ST3 = sum(T3); ST4 = sum(T4)
```

Then the variance for each study can be obtained as:

```
> Var.lnOddsRatio = 0.5*(
 (T1*T3)/ST3^2+(T1*T4+T2*T3)/(ST3*ST4)+T2*T4/ST4^2)
> Var.lnOddsRatio

[1] 0.000250 0.000338 0.000590 0.000672
```

And the variance for the log odds ratio is:

```
> Var.lnMH = sum(Var.lnOddsRatio)
> Var.lnMH

[1] 0.00185
```

With this variance, the 95% CI for the log odds ratio is:

```
> lowCI.lnMH = log(OR.MH)-1.96*sqrt(Var.lnMH)
> upCI.lnMH = log(OR.MH)+1.96*sqrt(Var.lnMH)
> cat("The 95% CI for log-MH =(", round(lowCI.lnMH, 4), ",",
 round(upCI.lnMH, 4), ")", sep="", "\n\n")

The 95% CI for log-MH =(-0.264,-0.0955)
```

Transforming back to the original scale, the 95% CI for the odds ratio is:

```
> lowCI.MH = exp(lowCI.lnMH)
> upCI.MH  = exp(upCI.lnMH)
> cat("The 95% CI for MH =(", round(lowCI.MH, 4), ",",
 round(upCI.MH, 4), ")", sep="", "\n\n")

The 95% CI for MH =(0.768,0.909)
```

4.2.4.3 Meta-Analysis Using R Library `Meta`

The implementation for MH OR method in R library can be done easily by calling function `metabin` as follows:

```
> # MH OR meta-analysis
> ORMH.Statin = metabin(evhigh,nhigh,evstd,nstd,studlab=Study,
                                   data=dat, method="MH", sm="OR")
> # print the summary
> summary(ORMH.Statin)

Number of studies combined: k=4
                        OR          95%-CI      z  p.value
Fixed effect model   0.835  [0.768; 0.909] -4.18 < 0.0001
Random effects model 0.835  [0.768; 0.909] -4.18 < 0.0001

Quantifying heterogeneity:
tau^2 < 0.0001; H = 1 [1; 1.58]; I^2 = 0% [0%; 59.7%]
Test of heterogeneity:
    Q d.f.  p.value
 1.14    3   0.7673

Details on meta-analytical method:
- Mantel-Haenszel method
```

Interested readers can check the results from `metabin` with the results from the previous section and find that they are exactly the same.

The forest plot can be shown as in Figure 4.4 as follows:

```
> forest(ORMH.Statin)
```

4.2.5 Peto's Meta-Analysis Method

4.2.5.1 Peto's Odds Ratio

Another alternative to the MH method in analyzing odds ratios is Peto's method (Yusuf et al., 1985). The Peto's odds ratio can be biased, especially when there is a substantial difference between treatment and control group sizes, but it performs well in many situations.

For each study i, the Peto's odds ratio is defined as:

$$\hat{\Psi}_i = exp\left(\frac{O_i - E_i}{V_i}\right) \tag{4.27}$$

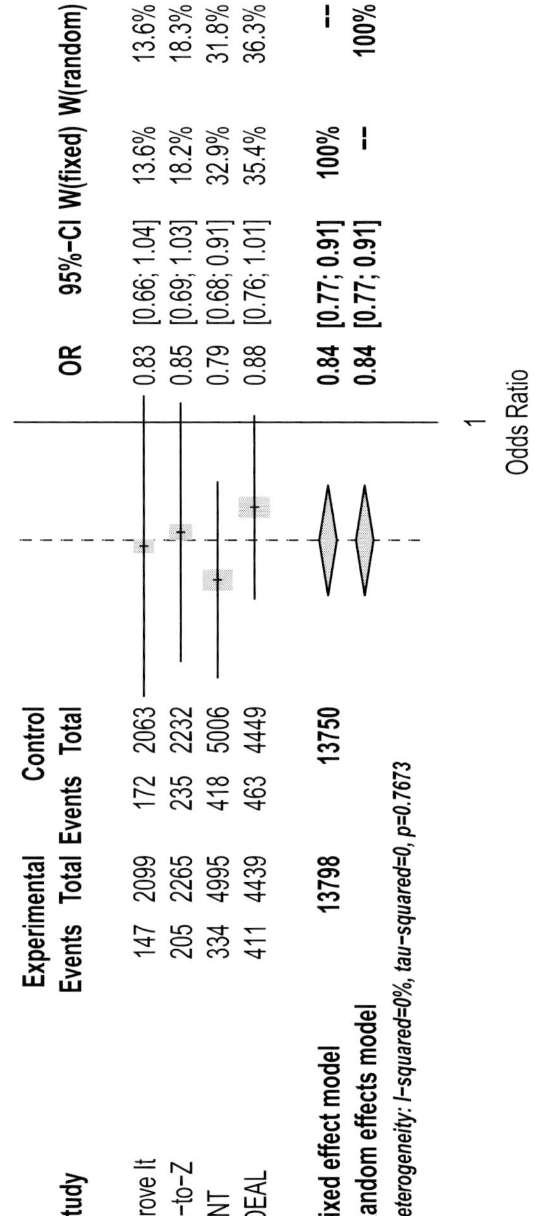

FIGURE 4.4: Meta-Analysis with Mantel-Haenszel Odds Ratio

where

$$
\begin{aligned}
O_i &= A_i \\
E_i &= \frac{(A_i + B_i)(A_i + C_i)}{N_i} \\
V_i &= \frac{(A_i + B_i)(C_i + D_i)(A_i + C_i)(B_i + D_i)}{N_i^2(N_i - 1)} \\
z_i &= \frac{O_i - E_i}{\sqrt{V_i}} \\
CI_i &= exp\left(\frac{(O_i - E_i) \pm z_{\alpha/2}\sqrt{V_i}}{V_i}\right)
\end{aligned}
$$

Note that O_i and E_i are the observed and expected counts in the ith 2 by 2 table. z_i is the asymptotically normal test statistic for the ith study, CI_i is the confidence interval where $z_{\alpha/2}$ as the quantile from the standard normal distribution. V_i is both the weighting factor and the variance for the difference between observed and expected $O_i - E_i$.

Then the pooled Peto's odds ratio is

$$
\Psi_{pooled} = exp\left(\frac{\sum_{i=1}^K (O_i - E_i)}{\sum_{i=1}^K V_i}\right) \tag{4.28}
$$

$$
CI_{pooled} = exp\left(\frac{\sum_{i=1}^K (O_i - E_i) \pm z_{\alpha/2}\sqrt{\sum_{i=1}^K V_i}}{\sum_{i=1}^K V_i}\right) \tag{4.29}
$$

4.2.5.2 Step by Step Implementation in R

First, the Peto's odds ratio for each study can be calculated as follows:

```
> # the needed quantities of observed and expected
> Oi   = A
> Ei   = (A+B)*(A+C)/N
> Vi   = (A+B)*(C+D)/N*(A+C)/N*(B+D)/(N-1)
```

Then the Peto's OR for each study can be calculated as:

```
> psii= exp( (Oi-Ei)/Vi)
> psii

[1] 0.828 0.846 0.787 0.879
```

and the CI for each study can then be computed as follows:

```
> # lower and upper CI bounds
> lowCIi = exp( (Oi-Ei-1.96*sqrt(Vi))/Vi )
> upCIi  = exp( (Oi-Ei + 1.96*sqrt(Vi))/Vi )
> lowCIi
[1] 0.659 0.695 0.679 0.764
> upCIi
[1] 1.041 1.030 0.913 1.010
```

Again we can see that only the third study is significant based on this CI approach. To perform the Peto's OR meta-analysis, we can calculate the pooled Peto's odds ratio for the entire study as follows:

```
> # pooled Peto's OR
> psi = exp( sum(Oi-Ei)/sum(Vi))
> psi

[1] 0.836

> # lower and upper CI bounds
> lowCI = exp( ( sum(Oi-Ei) - 1.96*sqrt(sum(Vi)))/sum(Vi) )
> upCI  = exp( ( sum(Oi-Ei) + 1.96*sqrt(sum(Vi)))/sum(Vi) )
> lowCI
[1] 0.768
> upCI
[1] 0.909
```

Again, this 95% CI does not cover zero concluding again that the experimental high-dose scheme is statistically more effective than the standard dose scheme.

As an exercise we encourage interested readers to compute the p-value and the (post) power for Peto's OR.

4.2.5.3 R Implementation in `meta`

The implementation of this Peto's OR meta-analysis in R library can be done easily as follows:

```
> # call "metabin" for Peto's OR
> ORPeto.Statin =
```

```
metabin(evhigh,nhigh,evstd,nstd,studlab=Study,
               data=dat, method="Peto", sm="OR")
> # print the summary
> summary(ORPeto.Statin)

Number of studies combined: k=4


                         OR          95%-CI     z  p.value
Fixed effect model    0.836  [0.768; 0.909] -4.18 < 0.0001
Random effects model 0.836  [0.768; 0.909] -4.18 < 0.0001

Quantifying heterogeneity:
tau^2 < 0.0001; H = 1 [1; 1.57]; I^2 = 0% [0%; 59.5%]

Test of heterogeneity:
    Q d.f.  p.value
 1.13    3   0.7692

Details on meta-analytical method:
- Peto's method
- DerSimonian-Laird estimator for tau^2
```

The forest plot can be shown as in Figure 4.5 as follows:

```
> forest(ORPeto.Statin)
```

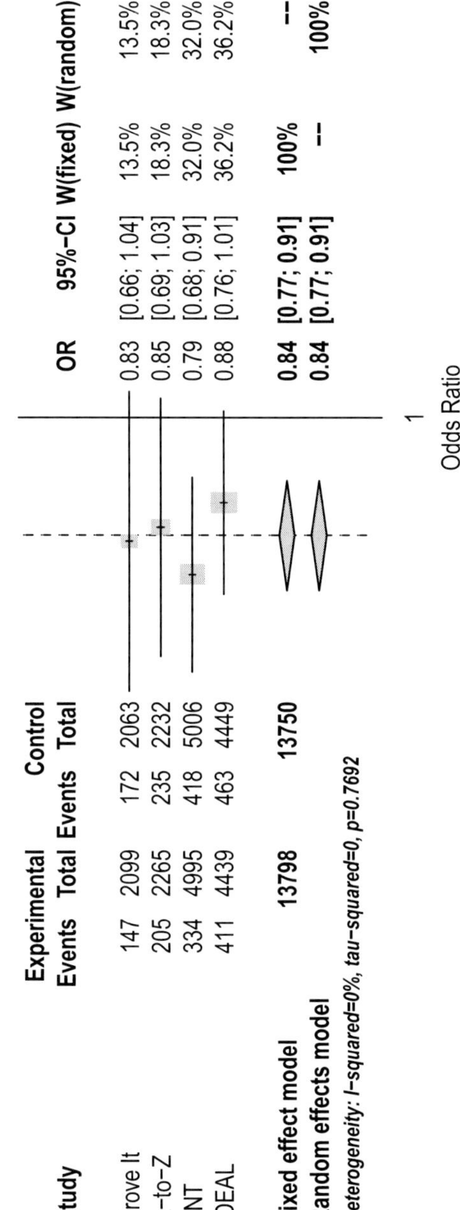

FIGURE 4.5: Meta-Analysis with Peto Odds Ratio

4.3 Meta-Analysis of Lamotrigine Studies

As shown in section 4.1.2, the data was read into R using `read.xls` and displayed in Table 4.2. The first category data can be printed using following R code:

```
> head(Lamo, n=10)

        Trial Events Total       Group Category
1  SCA100223     59   111 lamotrigine        1
2   SCA30924     47   131 lamotrigine        1
3   SCA40910     51   133 lamotrigine        1
4   SCAA2010     51   103 lamotrigine        1
5   SCAB2001     32    63 lamotrigine        1
6  SCA100223     44   109     placebo        1
7   SCA30924     37   128     placebo        1
8   SCA40910     39   124     placebo        1
9   SCAA2010     45   103     placebo        1
10  SCAB2001     21    66     placebo        1
```

4.3.1 Risk-Ratio

To reproduce the risk-ratio (RR) results in the Geddes et al.(2009) paper, we can call the `metabin` function for the category 1 data using following R code chunk as follows:

```
> # Get the Category 1 data
> d1     = Lamo[Lamo$Category==1,]
> evlamo = d1[d1$Group=="lamotrigine",]$Events
> nlamo  = d1[d1$Group=="lamotrigine",]$Total
> evcont = d1[d1$Group=="placebo",]$Events
> ncont  = d1[d1$Group=="placebo",]$Total
> trial  = d1[d1$Group=="placebo",]$Trial
> # Call metabin function for meta-analysis
> RR1.Lamo = metabin(evlamo,nlamo,evcont,ncont,studlab=trial,
```

```
label.e="Lamotrigine", label.c="Placebo", method="MH",
sm="RR")
> # print the RR fitting
> RR1.Lamo

                 RR          95%-CI %W(fixed) %W(random)
SCA100223 1.32  [0.988; 1.76]       23.6        26.4
SCA30924  1.24  [0.870; 1.77]       19.9        17.3
SCA40910  1.22  [0.870; 1.71]       21.5        19.1
SCAA2010  1.13  [0.845; 1.52]       24.0        25.3
SCAB2001  1.60  [1.040; 2.45]       10.9        11.9

Number of studies combined: k=5

                          RR         95%-CI    z  p.value
Fixed effect model    1.27  [1.09; 1.47] 3.13   0.0017
Random effects model 1.26  [1.09; 1.47] 3.12   0.0018

Quantifying heterogeneity:
tau^2 < 0.0001; H = 1 [1; 1.47]; I^2 = 0% [0%; 53.9%]

Test of heterogeneity:
   Q d.f. p.value
 1.8    4   0.772

Details on meta-analytical method:
- Mantel-Haenszel method
```

This reproduces all the results. The figure 1a in the paper can be produced simply using `forest` from the `meta` package as follows:

```
> forest(RR1.Lamo)
```

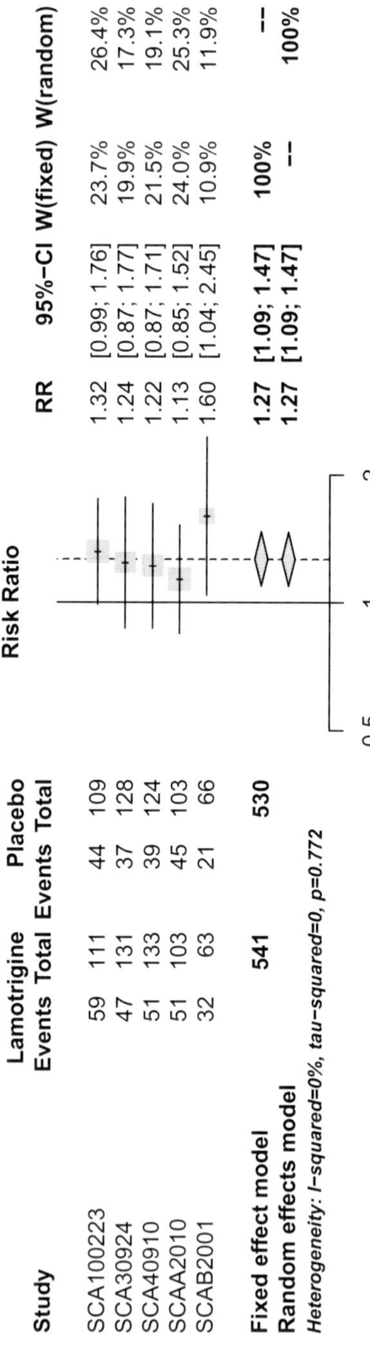

Study
Lamotrigine Events Total
Placebo Events Total
Risk Ratio
RR
95%−CI
W(fixed)
W(random)
SCA100223 59 111 44 109 1.32 [0.99; 1.76] 23.7% 26.4%
SCA30924 47 131 37 128 1.24 [0.87; 1.77] 19.9% 17.3%
SCA40910 51 133 39 124 1.22 [0.87; 1.71] 21.5% 19.1%
SCAA2010 51 103 45 103 1.13 [0.85; 1.52] 24.0% 25.3%
SCAB2001 32 63 21 66 1.60 [1.04; 2.45] 10.9% 11.9%
Fixed effect model 541 530 1.27 [1.09; 1.47] 100% --
Random effects model 1.27 [1.09; 1.47] -- 100%
Heterogeneity: I−squared=0%, tau−squared=0, p=0.772
0.5
1
2

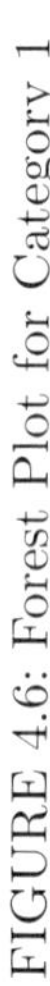
FIGURE 4.6: Forest Plot for Category 1

Similarly, the meta-analysis for > 50% reduction on MADRS (i.e. Category 2) can be done using the following R code chunk:

```
> # Get the Category 2 data
> d2     = Lamo[Lamo$Category==2,]
> evlamo = d2[d2$Group=="lamotrigine",]$Events
> nlamo  = d2[d2$Group=="lamotrigine",]$Total
> evcont = d2[d2$Group=="placebo",]$Events
> ncont  = d2[d2$Group=="placebo",]$Total
> trial  = d2[d2$Group=="placebo",]$Trial
> # Call metabin function for meta-analysis
> RR2.Lamo = metabin(evlamo,nlamo,evcont,ncont,studlab=trial,
 label.e="Lamotrigine", label.c="Placebo", method="MH",
 sm="RR")
> # print the RR fitting
> RR2.Lamo

            RR          95%-CI %W(fixed) %W(random)
SCA100223 1.32  [0.988; 1.76]     21.97      24.19
SCA30924  1.24  [0.911; 1.70]     22.02      20.68
SCA40910  1.09  [0.806; 1.48]     24.07      21.77
SCAA2010  1.11  [0.829; 1.48]     22.76      23.71
SCAB2001  1.71  [1.085; 2.69]      9.18       9.65

Number of studies combined: k=5

                       RR         95%-CI    z  p.value
Fixed effect model   1.24  [1.07; 1.42] 2.93   0.0034
Random effects model 1.23  [1.07; 1.42] 2.87   0.0041

Quantifying heterogeneity:
tau^2 < 0.0001; H = 1 [1; 2]; I^2 = 0% [0%; 75%]

Test of heterogeneity:
    Q d.f.  p.value
 3.33    4   0.5045
```

```
Details on meta-analytical method:
- Mantel-Haenszel method
```

In comparing these results with those in the paper, we see there is a slight discrepancy for study SCA100223. In the paper, the RR was reported as 1.26 with CI of (0.95, 1.67) whereas the results from R is 1.32 with CI of (0.99, 1.76). This may be a good exercise for the reader to investigate and explain the nature of the discrepancy. In addition, we do not produce Figure 2a in the paper since readers can reproduce it using `forest` as we did for Figure 4.6.

Categories 3 and 4 reflect subsets of category 2 based on the mean baseline HRSD score being < 24 or ≥ 24. The meta-analyses can be produced using the following R code chunks:

```
> # Get the Category 3 data
> d3      = Lamo[Lamo$Category==3,]
> evlamo = d3[d3$Group=="lamotrigine",]$Events
> nlamo  = d3[d3$Group=="lamotrigine",]$Total
> evcont = d3[d3$Group=="placebo",]$Events
> ncont  = d3[d3$Group=="placebo",]$Total
> trial  = d3[d3$Group=="placebo",]$Trial
> # Call metabin function for meta-analysis
> RR3.Lamo = metabin(evlamo,nlamo,evcont,ncont,studlab=trial,
 label.e="Lamotrigine", label.c="Placebo", method="MH",
 sm="RR")
> # print the RR fitting for Category 3
> RR3.Lamo

             RR          95%-CI %W(fixed) %W(random)
SCA100223 0.983  [0.659; 1.47]      20.6       18.9
SCA30924  1.174  [0.800; 1.72]      20.2       20.6
SCA40910  0.969  [0.665; 1.41]      25.1       21.3
SCAA2010  1.071  [0.763; 1.50]      22.8       26.2
SCAB2001  1.265  [0.781; 2.05]      11.3       13.0

Number of studies combined: k=5
```

```
                          RR           95%-CI      z  p.value
Fixed effect model    1.07  [0.899; 1.27] 0.764   0.445
Random effects model 1.07  [0.903; 1.28] 0.809   0.4185

Quantifying heterogeneity:
tau^2 < 0.0001; H = 1 [1; 1.16]; I^2 = 0% [0%; 26.2%]

Test of heterogeneity:
    Q d.f. p.value
 1.13    4    0.89

Details on meta-analytical method:
- Mantel-Haenszel method

> # Now analyze category 4
> # first get the Category 4 data
> d4     = Lamo[Lamo$Category==4,]
> evlamo = d4[d4$Group=="lamotrigine",]$Events
> nlamo  = d4[d4$Group=="lamotrigine",]$Total
> evcont = d4[d4$Group=="placebo",]$Events
> ncont  = d4[d4$Group=="placebo",]$Total
> trial  = d4[d4$Group=="placebo",]$Trial
> # Call metabin function for meta-analysis
> RR4.Lamo = metabin(evlamo,nlamo,evcont,ncont,studlab=trial,
 label.e="Lamotrigine", label.c="Placebo", method="MH",
 sm="RR")
> # print the RR fitting for Category 4
> RR4.Lamo

              RR          95%-CI %W(fixed) %W(random)
SCA100223 1.63  [1.065; 2.49]      25.78      30.75
SCA30924  1.33  [0.803; 2.21]      24.77      21.59
SCA40910  1.34  [0.804; 2.23]      21.78      21.25
SCAA2010  1.22  [0.721; 2.06]      21.56      20.03
SCAB2001  2.75  [1.082; 6.99]       6.12       6.38
```

```
Number of studies combined: k=5

                         RR         95%-CI    z  p.value
Fixed effect model   1.47  [1.16; 1.86] 3.22   0.0013
Random effects model 1.46  [1.15; 1.85] 3.15   0.0016

Quantifying heterogeneity:
tau^2 < 0.0001; H = 1 [1; 1.8]; I^2 = 0% [0%; 69.3%]

Test of heterogeneity:
    Q d.f.  p.value
 2.71    4   0.6076

Details on meta-analytical method:
- Mantel-Haenszel method
```

The same conclusions are produced where Lamotrigine was more beneficial than placebo in patients with severe depression at baseline but not in patients with moderate depression. We again encourage readers to reproduce Figure 2 in the paper by using `forest`.

We did the meta-analysis in this chapter using the Mantel- Haenszel weighting method (i.e. `method="MH"`) corresponding to the original paper. As an exercise, we encourage readers to use the inverse weighting (i.e. `method="Inverse"`) as an alternative meta-analysis.

4.3.2 Risk-Difference

Further analysis for this dataset can be performed using the risk-difference (RD) as the treatment effect. We can use `metabin` function and change summary method (i.e. `sm`) from `RR` to `RD`. In addition, we are going to replace the Mantel-Haenszel weighting scheme (i.e. `method="MH"`) with the inverse weighting scheme (i.e. `method="Inverse"`) in this analysis and leave the Mantel-Haenszel weighting scheme to interested readers (just replace `method="Inverse"` with `method="MH"`) as an exercise. We put all four categories into one R code chunk without producing the `forest`, but with detailed explanations in the code chunk as follows:

```
> #
> # meta-analysis for Category 1 HRSD data
> #
> evlamo = d1[d1$Group=="lamotrigine",]$Events
> nlamo  = d1[d1$Group=="lamotrigine",]$Total
> evcont = d1[d1$Group=="placebo",]$Events
> ncont  = d1[d1$Group=="placebo",]$Total
> trial  = d1[d1$Group=="placebo",]$Trial
> # Call metabin function for meta-analysis
> RD1.Lamo = metabin(evlamo,nlamo,evcont,ncont,studlab=trial,
        label.e="Lamotrigine", label.c="Placebo",
        method="Inverse", sm="RD")
> # print the result for category 1
> RD1.Lamo
```

```
              RD             95%-CI %W(fixed) %W(random)
SCA100223 0.1279  [-0.0029; 0.259]       19.5       19.5
SCA30924  0.0697  [-0.0439; 0.183]       25.8       25.8
SCA40910  0.0689  [-0.0473; 0.185]       24.7       24.7
SCAA2010  0.0583  [-0.0778; 0.194]       18.0       18.0
SCAB2001  0.1898  [ 0.0228; 0.357]       12.0       12.0

Number of studies combined: k=5

                          RD          95%-CI    z  p.value
Fixed effect model    0.0932 [0.0354;0.151] 3.16 0.0016
Random effects model  0.0932 [0.0354;0.151] 3.16 0.0016

Quantifying heterogeneity:
tau^2 < 0.0001; H = 1 [1; 1.6]; I^2 = 0% [0%; 61.1%]

Test of heterogeneity:
    Q d.f. p.value
```

```
 2.14    4    0.71

Details on meta-analytical method:
- Inverse variance method
- DerSimonian-Laird estimator for tau^2

> #
> # meta-analysis for Category 2 MADRS data
> #
> evlamo = d2[d2$Group=="lamotrigine",]$Events
> nlamo  = d2[d2$Group=="lamotrigine",]$Total
> evcont = d2[d2$Group=="placebo",]$Events
> ncont  = d2[d2$Group=="placebo",]$Total
> trial  = d2[d2$Group=="placebo",]$Trial
> # Call metabin function for meta-analysis
> RD2.Lamo = metabin(evlamo,nlamo,evcont,ncont,studlab=trial,
 label.e="Lamotrigine", label.c="Placebo", method="Inverse",
 sm="RD")
> # print the result for category 2
> RD2.Lamo

               RD              95%-CI %W(fixed) %W(random)
SCA100223 0.1279  [-0.0029; 0.259]       20.1        20.1
SCA30924  0.0837  [-0.0344; 0.202]       24.6        24.6
SCA40910  0.0345  [-0.0851; 0.154]       24.1        24.1
SCAA2010  0.0485  [-0.0876; 0.185]       18.5        18.5
SCAB2001  0.2042  [ 0.0393; 0.369]       12.6        12.6

Number of studies combined: k=5

                           RD          95%-CI    z  p.value
Fixed effect model    0.0895 [0.0308;0.148] 2.99 0.0028
Random effects model 0.0895 [0.0308;0.148] 2.99 0.0028

Quantifying heterogeneity:
tau^2 < 0.0001; H = 1 [1; 2.01]; I^2 = 0% [0%; 75.2%]
```

```
Test of heterogeneity:
    Q d.f.  p.value
 3.36    4   0.4996

Details on meta-analytical method:
- Inverse variance method
- DerSimonian-Laird estimator for tau^2

> #
> # meta-analysis for category 3
> # i.e. moderate depressed individuals at baseline
> #
> evlamo = d3[d3$Group=="lamotrigine",]$Events
> nlamo  = d3[d3$Group=="lamotrigine",]$Total
> evcont = d3[d3$Group=="placebo",]$Events
> ncont  = d3[d3$Group=="placebo",]$Total
> trial  = d3[d3$Group=="placebo",]$Trial
> # Call metabin function for meta-analysis
> RD3.Lamo = metabin(evlamo,nlamo,evcont,ncont,studlab=trial,
 label.e="Lamotrigine", label.c="Placebo", method="Inverse",
 sm="RD")
> # print the result for category 3
> RD3.Lamo

                RD             95%-CI %W(fixed) %W(random)
SCA100223 -0.0076  [-0.1842; 0.169]      20.4        20.4
SCA30924   0.0730  [-0.0998; 0.246]      21.3        21.3
SCA40910  -0.0125  [-0.1638; 0.139]      27.8        27.8
SCAA2010   0.0369  [-0.1446; 0.218]      19.3        19.3
SCAB2001   0.1198  [-0.1201; 0.360]      11.1        11.1

Number of studies combined: k=5

                         RD           95%-CI     z p.value
Fixed effect model   0.0309 [-0.0489;0.111] 0.759 0.4476
```

```
Random effects model 0.0309 [-0.0489;0.111] 0.759 0.4476

Quantifying heterogeneity:
tau^2 < 0.0001; H = 1 [1; 1.23]; I^2 = 0% [0%; 33.9%]

Test of heterogeneity:
    Q d.f.  p.value
 1.26    4   0.8684

Details on meta-analytical method:
- Inverse variance method
- DerSimonian-Laird estimator for tau^2

> #
> # meta-analysis for category 4:
> #        i.e. severe depressed individuals at baseline
> #
> evlamo = d4[d4$Group=="lamotrigine",]$Events
> nlamo  = d4[d4$Group=="lamotrigine",]$Total
> evcont = d4[d4$Group=="placebo",]$Events
> ncont  = d4[d4$Group=="placebo",]$Total
> trial  = d4[d4$Group=="placebo",]$Trial
> # Call metabin function for meta-analysis
> RD4.Lamo = metabin(evlamo,nlamo,evcont,ncont,studlab=trial,
 label.e="Lamotrigine", label.c="Placebo", method="Inverse",
 sm="RD")
> # print the result for category 4
> RD4.Lamo

              RD               95%-CI %W(fixed) %W(random)
SCA100223 0.2433  [ 0.0502; 0.436]       19.2       19.2
SCA30924  0.0909  [-0.0672; 0.249]       28.6       28.6
SCA40910  0.1135  [-0.0814; 0.308]       18.9       18.9
SCAA2010  0.0767  [-0.1240; 0.277]       17.8       17.8
SCAB2001  0.2500  [ 0.0351; 0.465]       15.5       15.5
```

```
Number of studies combined: k=5

                          RD           95%-CI    z  p.value
Fixed effect model    0.147  [0.062; 0.231] 3.39   0.0007
Random effects model 0.147  [0.062; 0.231] 3.39   0.0007

Quantifying heterogeneity:
tau^2 < 0.0001; H = 1 [1; 1.87]; I^2 = 0% [0%; 71.4%]

Test of heterogeneity:
    Q d.f.  p.value
 2.91    4   0.5737

Details on meta-analytical method:
- Inverse variance method
- DerSimonian-Laird estimator for tau^2
```

From the outputs, we see that with the exception of study SCAB2001, the first four studies (i.e. SCA100223, SCA30924, SCA40910, SCAA2010) have a 95% CI covering zero for all four categories indicating that lamotrigine was not more beneficial than the placebo if analyzed individually. However, when combined, a statistically significant result is found for categories of 1,2, and 4. This result is similar to the finding from RR indicated in the previous section as well as in the Geddes et al. paper.

In this analysis of RD, both the fixed-effects and random- effects meta-analysis gave same results because of statistically insignificant heterogeneity as seen from the Q-statistic with estimated between-study variance $\hat{\tau}^2 = 0$.

4.3.3 Odds Ratio

Odds ratio (OR) is a commonly used metric in the analysis of binomial data. We illustrate the meta-analysis using OR for the lamotrigine data. There are several methods implemented for OR in the R package `meta` as described in Section 4.2. To control the number of pages in this chapter, we only illustrate the Mantel-Haenszel weighting scheme (i.e., `method="MH"`) here, and leave the inverse weighting scheme (i.e. `method="Inverse"`) and the Peto's method (i.e., method="Peto") to interested readers as exercises. In addition, we encourage readers to produce the forest plots for each analysis.

The implementation of the OR with Mantel-Haenszel weighting scheme can be done with the following code chunk:

```
> #
> # meta-analysis for Category 1 HRSD data
> #
> evlamo = d1[d1$Group=="lamotrigine",]$Events
> nlamo  = d1[d1$Group=="lamotrigine",]$Total
> evcont = d1[d1$Group=="placebo",]$Events
> ncont  = d1[d1$Group=="placebo",]$Total
> trial  = d1[d1$Group=="placebo",]$Trial
> # Call metabin function for meta-analysis
> OR1.Lamo = metabin(evlamo,nlamo,evcont,ncont,studlab=trial,
 label.e="Lamotrigine", label.c="Placebo", method="MH",
 sm="OR")
> # print the result for category 1
> OR1.Lamo

           OR         95%-CI %W(fixed) %W(random)
SCA100223 1.68  [0.982; 2.86]     20.29       21.6
SCA30924  1.38  [0.816; 2.32]     23.41       22.6
SCA40910  1.36  [0.809; 2.27]     24.28       23.2
SCAA2010  1.26  [0.731; 2.19]     22.16       20.5
SCAB2001  2.21  [1.081; 4.53]      9.85       12.0

Number of studies combined: k=5

                       OR         95%-CI    z  p.value
Fixed effect model   1.49   [1.16; 1.91] 3.15   0.0016
Random effects model 1.49   [1.16; 1.91] 3.14   0.0017

Quantifying heterogeneity:
tau^2 < 0.0001; H = 1 [1; 1.52]; I^2 = 0% [0%; 56.7%]
```

```
Test of heterogeneity:
    Q d.f.  p.value
 1.92    4   0.7504

Details on meta-analytical method:
- Mantel-Haenszel method

> #
> # meta-analysis for Category 2 MADRS data
> #
> evlamo = d2[d2$Group=="lamotrigine",]$Events
> nlamo  = d2[d2$Group=="lamotrigine",]$Total
> evcont = d2[d2$Group=="placebo",]$Events
> ncont  = d2[d2$Group=="placebo",]$Total
> trial  = d2[d2$Group=="placebo",]$Trial
> # Call metabin function for meta-analysis
> OR2.Lamo = metabin(evlamo,nlamo,evcont,ncont,studlab=trial,
 label.e="Lamotrigine", label.c="Placebo", method="MH",
 sm="OR")
> # print the result for category 2
> OR2.Lamo

            OR          95%-CI %W(fixed) %W(random)
SCA100223 1.68  [0.982; 2.86]     19.36       21.0
SCA30924  1.43  [0.862; 2.36]     23.71       23.7
SCA40910  1.16  [0.700; 1.91]     26.55       23.9
SCAA2010  1.22  [0.703; 2.10]     21.61       20.0
SCAB2001  2.40  [1.159; 4.96]      8.77       11.4

Number of studies combined: k=5

                       OR         95%-CI    z  p.value
Fixed effect model   1.44  [1.13; 1.84] 2.94   0.0033
Random effects model 1.44  [1.13; 1.84] 2.92   0.0035

Quantifying heterogeneity:
```

```
tau^2 < 0.0001; H = 1 [1; 2]; I^2 = 0% [0%; 74.9%]

Test of heterogeneity:
    Q d.f. p.value
 3.31    4   0.507

Details on meta-analytical method:
- Mantel-Haenszel method

> #
> # meta-analysis for category 3:
> #         (moderate depressed individuals at baseline)
> #
> evlamo = d3[d3$Group=="lamotrigine",]$Events
> nlamo  = d3[d3$Group=="lamotrigine",]$Total
> evcont = d3[d3$Group=="placebo",]$Events
> ncont  = d3[d3$Group=="placebo",]$Total
> trial  = d3[d3$Group=="placebo",]$Trial
> # Call metabin function for meta-analysis
> OR3.Lamo = metabin(evlamo,nlamo,evcont,ncont,studlab=trial,
 label.e="Lamotrigine", label.c="Placebo", method="MH",
 sm="OR")
> # print the result for category 3
> OR3.Lamo

             OR          95%-CI %W(fixed) %W(random)
SCA100223 0.970  [0.474; 1.98]     22.26       20.7
SCA30924  1.343  [0.666; 2.71]     19.77       21.6
SCA40910  0.949  [0.506; 1.78]     29.12       26.8
SCAA2010  1.160  [0.559; 2.41]     19.55       19.8
SCAB2001  1.619  [0.611; 4.29]      9.31       11.2

Number of studies combined: k=5

                      OR          95%-CI     z  p.value
Fixed effect model   1.14  [0.82; 1.57] 0.765   0.4444
```

```
Random effects model 1.13  [0.82; 1.57] 0.762   0.446

Quantifying heterogeneity:
tau^2 < 0.0001; H = 1 [1; 1.22]; I^2 = 0% [0%; 32.4%]

Test of heterogeneity:
    Q d.f. p.value
 1.23    4   0.873

Details on meta-analytical method:
- Mantel-Haenszel method

> #
> # meta-analysis for category 4:
> #   (severe depressed individuals at baseline)
> #
> evlamo = d4[d4$Group=="lamotrigine",]$Events
> nlamo  = d4[d4$Group=="lamotrigine",]$Total
> evcont = d4[d4$Group=="placebo",]$Events
> ncont  = d4[d4$Group=="placebo",]$Total
> trial  = d4[d4$Group=="placebo",]$Trial
> # Call metabin function for meta-analysis
> OR4.Lamo = metabin(evlamo,nlamo,evcont,ncont,studlab=trial,
 label.e="Lamotrigine", label.c="Placebo", method="MH",
 sm="OR")
> # print the result for category 4
> OR4.Lamo

            OR          95%-CI %W(fixed) %W(random)
SCA100223 2.70  [1.188;  6.13]     17.86      21.77
SCA30924  1.52  [0.728;  3.19]     29.48      26.90
SCA40910  1.62  [0.704;  3.71]     22.54      21.22
SCAA2010  1.38  [0.589;  3.24]     23.17      20.15
SCAB2001  3.88  [1.154; 13.06]      6.95       9.96

Number of studies combined: k=5
```

```
                        OR          95%-CI    z  p.value
Fixed effect model    1.89  [1.29; 2.76] 3.27   0.0011
Random effects model 1.88  [1.28; 2.76] 3.23   0.0012

Quantifying heterogeneity:
tau^2 < 0.0001; H = 1 [1; 1.92]; I^2 = 0% [0%; 72.8%]

Test of heterogeneity:
    Q d.f.  p.value
 3.06    4   0.5482

Details on meta-analytical method:
- Mantel-Haenszel method
```

Again, the results from the analyses of OR are similar to those of RR and of RD, further confirming that lamotrigine was statistically better than the placebo in treating bipolar depression.

4.4 Discussion

In this chapter, we illustrated meta-analysis methods for binomial data using published results from two clinical trials programs. The first dataset was from clinical trials designed to compare intensive statin therapy to moderate statin therapy in the reduction of cardiovascular outcomes. The other dataset was from clinical trials of lamotrigine designed for treating depression in patients with bipolar disorder. Both datasets were used to illustrate meta-analyses using the R package `meta`. The cardiovascular dataset was used primarily to illustrate meta-analysis methods with step-by-step implementation in R along with the mathematical formula as discussed in Section 4.2. The lamotrigine dataset further illustrated the R implementation in package `meta`.

For studies with binary or binomial outcome measures, we focused on the most commonly used measures of treatment effect: i.e risk difference (RD), risk ratio (RR) and odds ratio (OR). Thc arcsine (AS) difference can also be used as a measure of treatment effect, although it rarely appears in the medical literature. It is implemented in R package `meta` as `sm="AS"` as one of the summary methods. As discussed in Rucker et al. (2009), the `AS` has considerable promise in handling zeros and its asymptotic variance does not depend on the event probability. We encourage interested readers to experiment with `sm="AS"` for their own data.

Chapter 5

Meta-Analysis for Continuous Data

Continuous data are commonly reported as endpoints in clinical trials and other studies. In this chapter, we discuss the meta-analysis methods for this type of data. For continuous data, the typical reported summary statistics are the means and standard deviations (or standard errors along with the sample sizes).

Meta-analyses of means for continuous data are usually performed on the mean differences across studies in reference to the pooled variance. Similarly to Chapter 4, we introduce two published datasets in Section 5.1 and then describe the meta-analysis models to facilitate analyses in Section 5.2. Step-by-step R implementation of the methods are presented using the first dataset. The second dataset is used in Section 5.3 to illustrate the application of R package `meta` corresponding to the meta-analysis methods detailed in Section 5.2. Discussion appears in Section 5.4.

Note to readers: You need to install R packages `gdata` to read in the Excel data file, and `meta` to perform the meta-analysis.

5.1 Two Published Datasets

5.1.1 Impact of Intervention

Table 5.1 is reproduced from Table 14.1 in Borenstein et al. (2009). Interested readers can refer to the book for details. In this chapter, we use this dataset to illustrate the step-by-step calculations using R for continuous data methods.

TABLE 5.1: Impact of Intervention: Continuous Data

	Treated			Control		
Study	mean	SD	N	mean	SD	N
Carroll	94	22	60	92	20	60
Grant	98	21	65	92	22	65
Peck	98	28	40	88	26	40
Donat	94	19	200	82	17	200
Stewart	98	21	50	88	22	45
Young	96	21	85	92	22	85

5.1.2 Tubeless vs Standard Percutaneous Nephrolithotomy

To systematically review and compare tubeless percutaneous nephrolithotomy (PCNL) with standard PCNL for stones of the kidney or upper ureter, Wang et al. (2011) conducted a meta-analysis from all English language literature on studies from randomized controlled trials to obtain definitive conclusions for clinical practice. The paper can be accessed from `http://www.ncbi.nlm.nih.gov/pubmed/21883839`.

The authors found 127 studies from the first search. After initial screening of the title and abstract, 20 studies met the inclusion criteria. Upon further screening the full text of these 20 studies, 7 studies were included in their meta-analysis. To reproduce the results from this paper, we entered all the data from these 7 studies into the excel databook `dat4Meta` which can be loaded into R using following R code chunk:

```
> # Load the library
> require(gdata)
> # Get the data path
> datfile = "Your Data Path/dat4Meta.xls"
> # Call "read.xls" to read the Excel data
> dat  = read.xls(datfile, sheet="Data_tubeless",
                  perl="c:/perl64/bin/perl.exe")
```

The dataset can be seen in Table 5.2. Note that in this table, column `Outcome` lists the four outcome measures considered in the paper which are: operation duration (abbreviated by "duration"), length of hospital stay (abbreviated by "LOS"), analgesic requirement after tubeless (abbreviated by "analgesic") and the pre- and post-operative hematocrit changes (abbreviated by "hematocrit"). Column `Study` denotes the selected clinical studies for this meta-analysis. The remaining columns: `Mean.E`, `SD.E`, `n.E`, `Mean.C`, `SD.C` and `n.C` denote the means, standard deviations and total observations from the experimental and control arms, respectively.

The authors performed their meta-analysis using the Cochrane Review Manager (REVMAN 5.0) software. In this chapter, we use the R package `meta` to re-analyze this dataset.

TABLE 5.2: Data from PCNL Studies

Outcome	Study	Mean.E	SD.E	n.E	Mean.C	SD.C	n.C
duration	Ahmet Tefekli 2007	60	9	17	76	10	18
duration	B.Lojanapiwat 2010	49	24	45	57	20	59
duration	Hemendra N. Shah 2008	51	10	33	47	16	32
duration	Hemendra Shah 2009	52	23	454	68	34	386
duration	J. Jun-Ou 2010	47	17	43	59	18	52
duration	Michael Choi 2006	82	18	12	73	15	12
LOS	Ahmet Tefekli 2007	38	10	17	67	22	18
LOS	B.Lojanapiwat 2010	85	23	45	129	54	59
LOS	Hemendra N. Shah 2008	35	11	33	44	22	32
LOS	Hemendra Shah 2009	34	17	454	56	62	386
LOS	J. Jun-Ou 2010	82	24	43	106	35	52
LOS	Madhu S. Agrawal 2008	22	4	101	54	5	101
LOS	Michael Choi 2006	37	24	12	38	24	12
analgesic	B.Lojanapiwat 2010	39	35	45	75	32	59
analgesic	Hemendra N. Shah 2008	150	97	33	246	167	32
analgesic	Hemendra Shah 2009	103	116	454	250	132	386
analgesic	J. Jun-Ou 2010	37	31	43	70	36	52
analgesic	Madhu S. Agrawal 2008	82	24	101	126	33	101
haematocrit	Ahmet Tefekli 2007	2	1	17	1	0	18
haematocrit	Hemendra N. Shah 2008	0	0	33	0	1	32
haematocrit	Hemendra Shah 2009	1	1	454	1	2	386
haematocrit	Madhu S. Agrawal 2008	0	0	101	0	0	202

5.2 Methods for Continuous Data

First suppose that the objective of a study is to compare two groups, such as Treated (referenced as 1) and Control (referenced as 2), in terms of their means. Let μ_1 and μ_2 be the true (population) means of the two groups. The population mean difference is defined as

$$\Delta = \mu_1 - \mu_2 \tag{5.1}$$

and the standardized mean difference

$$\delta = \frac{\mu_1 - \mu_2}{\sigma} \tag{5.2}$$

which is usually used as the effect size.

5.2.1 Estimate the Mean Difference Δ

For multiple studies that report outcome measures in the same scales or units, a meta-analysis can be carried out directly on the differences in means and preserve the original scales. In this situation, all calculations are relatively straightforward. For each study, we estimate Δ directly from the reported means as follows. Let $\bar{X}_1$ and $\bar{X}_2$ be the reported sample means of the two groups. Then the estimate of the population mean difference Δ is the difference in sample means:

$$D = \hat{\Delta} = \bar{X}_1 - \bar{X}_2 \tag{5.3}$$

For further statistical inference, we need to calculate the standard deviation of D which is easily done from the reported sample standard errors from the study. Let S_1 and S_2, n_1 and n_2, denote the corresponding sample standard errors and sample sizes in the two groups. Then the variance of D can be obtained as:

$$V_D = \frac{S_1^2}{n_1} + \frac{S_2^2}{n_2}, \tag{5.4}$$

if we do not assume homogeneity of variances for the two groups, i,e. $\sigma_1 \neq \sigma_2$. With the assumption of homogeneity of variance (i.e. $\sigma_1 = \sigma_2 = \sigma$) in the two groups, the variance of D is calculated using the pooled sample variance as:

$$V_D = \frac{n_1 + n_2}{n_1 n_2} S_{pooled}^2, \tag{5.5}$$

where

$$S_{pooled} = \sqrt{\frac{(n_1 - 1)S_1^2 + (n_2 - 1)S_2^2}{n_1 + n_2 - 2}}. \tag{5.6}$$

In either case, the standard deviation of D can be obtained by the square root of V_D as:

$$SE_D = \sqrt{V_D}. \tag{5.7}$$

Meta-analysis would then proceed by combining the differences (Ds) in sample means of the two groups across the individual studies and using the appropriate function of the variances (V_D) for statistical inference.

5.2.2 Estimate the Standardized Mean Difference δ

When different measurement scales (for example, different instruments in different laboratories or different clinical sites) are used in individual studies, it is meaningless to try to combine mean differences in the original scales using meta-analysis techniques. In such cases, a meaningful measure to be used for meta-analysis is the standardized mean difference δ as suggested by Cohen (1988) as the effect size in statistical power analysis.

Again, denote the population means of two groups by μ_1 and μ_2 and their corresponding variances by σ_1^2 and σ_2^2, respectively. Then the standardized mean difference or effect size (ES) δ is defined as the difference between μ_1 and μ_2 divided by their standard deviation which is denoted by

$$\delta = \frac{\mu_1 - \mu_2}{\sigma} \tag{5.8}$$

where σ is the associated standard deviation from either the population control group or a pooled population standard deviation.

To estimate the ES of δ, two commonly proposed measures are as follows. One of the measures is the known as Cohen's d (Cohen, 1988) and is given by:

$$d = \frac{\bar{X}_1 - \bar{X}_2}{S} \tag{5.9}$$

where the standardized quantity S is the pooled sample standard error as $S = \sqrt{S^2}$ where

$$S^2 = \frac{(n_1 - 1)S_1^2 + (n_2 - 1)S_2^2}{n_1 + n_2}.$$

The second measure of δ is known as Hedges' g (Hedges, 1982) defined as

$$g = \frac{\bar{X}_1 - \bar{X}_2}{S^*} \tag{5.10}$$

where

$$S^{*2} = \frac{(n_1 - 1)S_1^2 + (n_2 - 1)S_2^2}{n_1 + n_2 - 2}.$$

It is shown in Hedges and Olkin (1985) that

$$E(g) \approx \delta + \frac{3\delta}{4N - 9} \tag{5.11}$$

$$Var(g) \approx \frac{1}{\tilde{n}} + \frac{\delta^2}{2(N - 3.94)} \tag{5.12}$$

where

$$N = n_1 + n_2,\ \tilde{n} = \frac{n_1 n_2}{n_1 + n_2}$$

With the assumptions of equal variances in both groups and normality of the data, Hedges (1981) showed that $\sqrt{\tilde{n}}g$ follows a noncentral t-distribution with noncentrality parameter $\sqrt{\tilde{n}}\theta$ and $n_1 + n_2 - 2$ degrees of freedom. Based on this conclusion, the exact mean and variance of Hedges' g are given by

$$E(g) = \sqrt{\frac{N-2}{2}}\frac{\Gamma[(N-3)/2]}{\Gamma[(N-2)/2]}\delta \tag{5.13}$$

$$Var(g) = \frac{N-2}{N-4}(1+\delta^2) - \delta^2 \frac{N-2}{2}\frac{\{\Gamma[(N-3)/2]\}^2}{\{\Gamma[(N-2)/2]\}^2} \tag{5.14}$$

where $\Gamma()$ is the gamma function.

It should be noted that g is *biased* as an estimator for the population effect size δ. However, this bias can be easily corrected by multiplication with a factor since the exact mean in equation (5.13) is well approximated by equation (5.11) so that an approximately unbiased standardized mean difference g^* is given by

$$g^* \approx \left(1 - \frac{3}{4N - 9}\right) g = J \times g \tag{5.15}$$

It can be seen that the correction factor J above is always less than 1 which would lead to g^* always being less than g in absolute value. However J will be very close to 1 when N is large.

We denoted this unbiased estimator as g^* in this book to avoid confusion. Confusion about the notations has resulted since Hedges and Olkin (1985) in their seminal book referred to this unbiased estimator as d, which is not the same as Cohen's d.

With this unbiased form of g^*, the estimated variance is approximated using equation (5.12) as follows:

$$\widehat{Var}(g^*) \approx \frac{1}{\tilde{n}} + \frac{g^{*2}}{2(N-3.94)} \tag{5.16}$$

For statistical inference of ES δ for $H_0 : \delta = 0$ versus $H_1 : \delta \neq 0$ based on Hedges g, the typical standardized normal statistic can be constructed as follows:

$$Z = \frac{\hat{\hat{\delta}}}{\widehat{Var}(\hat{\delta})} = \frac{g^*}{\widehat{Var}(g^*)} \tag{5.17}$$

where g^* is from equation (5.11) and $\widehat{Var}(g^*)$ is from equation (5.16). H_0 is rejected if $|Z|$ exceeds $z_{\alpha/2}$, the upper $\alpha/2$ cut-off point of the standard normal distribution. A confidence interval for δ can be constructed as

$$1-\alpha \approx Pr\left[g^* - z_{\alpha/2}\sqrt{\widehat{Var}(g^*)} \leq \delta \leq g^* + z_{\alpha/2}\sqrt{\widehat{Var}(g^*)}\right]. \tag{5.18}$$

Note that the Cohen's d in equation (5.9) is proportional to Hedges' g in equation (5.10) as

$$d = \frac{n_1+n_2}{n_1+n_2-2}g = \frac{n_1+n_2}{n_1+n_2-2}\frac{g^*}{J}. \tag{5.19}$$

The results from Hedges g can be easily transformed to provide the mean and variance of Cohen's d.

Readers may be aware that there are several slightly different calculations for the variance of g in the literature. We used (5.16) to comply with the R `meta` package. In Borenstein et al. (2009), $2N$, instead of $2(N-3.94)$, is used at the denominator of the second term of the variance formula (5.16). Another commonly used alternative is $2(N-2)$. All these calculations are almost identical in practice unless n_1 and n_2 are very small which is usually not the case in meta-analysis.

5.2.3 Step-by-Step Implementation in R

To illustrate the methods in this section for continuous data, we made use of the impact of intervention data from Borenstein et al. (2009) as seen in Table 5.1.

The estimation using Δ for the mean difference as discussed in section 5.2.1 is straightforward and is left to interested readers. We illustrate Hedges' method in this subsection for the standardized mean difference as seen in section 5.2.2.

5.2.3.1 Load the Data Into R

Since this is a small dataset, we will type the data into R as follows:

```
> # Type the data
> Carroll = c(94, 22,60,92, 20,60)
> Grant   = c(98, 21,65, 92,22, 65)
> Peck    = c(98, 28, 40,88 ,26, 40)
> Donat   = c( 94,19, 200, 82,17, 200)
> Stewart = c( 98, 21,50, 88,22 , 45)
> Young   = c(96,21,85, 92 ,22, 85)
> # Make a data frame
> dat     = as.data.frame(rbind(Carroll, Grant, Peck,
                                Donat, Stewart,Young))
> colnames(dat) = c("m.t","sd.t","n.t","m.c","sd.c","n.c")
> # Print the data
> dat
```

```
        m.t sd.t n.t m.c sd.c n.c
Carroll  94   22  60  92   20  60
Grant    98   21  65  92   22  65
Peck     98   28  40  88   26  40
Donat    94   19 200  82   17 200
Stewart  98   21  50  88   22  45
Young    96   21  85  92   22  85
```

5.2.3.2 Meta-Analysis using R Library meta

We first illustrate the application using R library `meta` with a simple code `metacont`. To do this, we first load the library as:

```
> library(meta)
```

Since the data are continuous, we call the R function `metacont` for this meta-analysis using the build-in summary function (`sm`) of `SMD` (i.e. standardized mean difference) with Hedges' adjusted g. The R code chunk is as follows:

```
> # call the metacont
> mod = metacont(n.t,m.t,sd.t,n.c,m.c,sd.c,
         data=dat,studlab=rownames(dat),sm="SMD")
> # print the meta-analysis
> mod
```

```
           SMD              95%-CI %W(fixed) %W(random)
Carroll 0.0945  [-0.2635; 0.453]      12.39       15.8
Grant   0.2774  [-0.0681; 0.623]      13.30       16.3
Peck    0.3665  [-0.0756; 0.809]       8.13       12.6
Donat   0.6644  [ 0.4630; 0.866]      39.16       23.3
Stewart 0.4618  [ 0.0535; 0.870]       9.53       13.8
Young   0.1852  [-0.1161; 0.486]      17.49       18.3

Number of studies combined: k=6

                       SMD          95%-CI    z  p.value
Fixed effect model   0.415  [0.289; 0.541] 6.45 < 0.0001
Random effects model 0.358  [0.152; 0.565] 3.40   0.0007

Quantifying heterogeneity:
tau^2 = 0.0372; H = 1.54 [1; 2.43]; I^2 = 58% [0%; 83%]

Test of heterogeneity:
     Q d.f. p.value
 11.91    5   0.036

Details on meta-analytical method:
- Inverse variance method
- DerSimonian-Laird estimator for tau^2
```

Notice that by changing `sm="MD"` in the above code chunk, the simple mean difference Δ in section 5.2.1 is obtained. We leave this as practice for interested readers.

The forest plot as seen in Figure 5.1 can be generated by calling `forest` as follows:

```
> forest(mod)
```

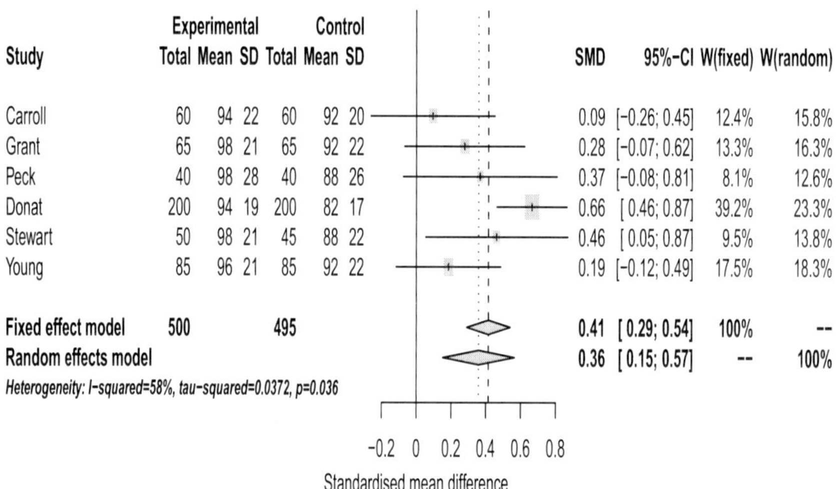

FIGURE 5.1: Forest Plot for the Continuous Data

5.2.3.3 Step-by-Step Calculations in R

To add to the understanding of the methods in this section, we make use of R to illustrate the step-by-step calculations to check against the output from subsection 5.2.3.2.

The first step in pooling the studies is to calculate the pooled variance or the standard deviation:

```
> # First get the pooled sd to calculate the SMD
> pooled.sd = sqrt(((dat$n.t-1)*dat$sd.t^2
          +(dat$n.c-1)*dat$sd.c^2)/(dat$n.t+dat$n.c-2))
> # Print the SD
> pooled.sd
```

```
[1] 21.0 21.5 27.0 18.0 21.5 21.5
```

With the pooled SD, we then calculate the standardized mean difference (SMD) as:

```
> # The standardized mean difference(SMD)
> g = (dat$m.t-dat$m.c)/pooled.sd
> # Print the SMD
> g
```

```
[1] 0.0951 0.2790 0.3701 0.6656 0.4656 0.1860
```

Since this SMD is biased, Hedges' correction should be used to adjust for this bias. The correction factor is calculated as follows:

```
> # Hedges correction factor
> N = dat$n.t+dat$n.c
> J = 1- 3/(4*N-9)
> # Print the correction factor J
> J
```

```
[1] 0.994 0.994 0.990 0.998 0.992 0.996
```

We see that these values are very close to 1. With these correction factors, we adjust the SMD for Hedges' g as follows:

```
> # now the Hedges g*
> gstar = J*g
> # Print it
> gstar
```

```
[1] 0.0945 0.2774 0.3665 0.6644 0.4618 0.1852
```

The variance for g^* is calculated as follows:

```
> # Variance of SMD
> var.gstar = (dat$n.t+dat$n.c)/(dat$n.t*dat$n.c)
>                 + gstar^2/(2*(dat$n.t+dat$n.c-3.94))

[1] 3.85e-05 3.05e-04 8.83e-04 5.57e-04 1.17e-03 1.03e-04

> # Print it
> var.gstar

[1] 0.0333 0.0308 0.0500 0.0100 0.0422 0.0235
```

Therefore the 95% CI for the 6 studies is constructed as:

```
> lowCI.gstar = gstar-1.96*sqrt(var.gstar)
> upCI.gstar  = gstar+1.96*sqrt(var.gstar)
> # Print the CIs and the SMD
> cbind(lowCI.gstar, gstar, upCI.gstar)

     lowCI.gstar  gstar upCI.gstar
[1,]     -0.2633 0.0945      0.452
[2,]     -0.0665 0.2774      0.621
[3,]     -0.0717 0.3665      0.805
[4,]      0.4684 0.6644      0.860
[5,]      0.0591 0.4618      0.865
[6,]     -0.1155 0.1852      0.486
```

Readers can check these results with the output from R `meta` and should find that they are exactly the same.

To combine the studies with fixed-effects model, we first calculate the weights as:

```
> # The individual weight
> w = 1/var.gstar
> w

[1]  30.0  32.5  20.0 100.0  23.7  42.5

> # The total weight
> tot.w = sum(w)
> tot.w
```

```
[1] 249

> # And the relative weight
> rel.w = w/tot.w
> rel.w

[1] 0.1206 0.1307 0.0804 0.4021 0.0952 0.1709
```

With these weights, we calculate the meta-estimate as:

```
> # Meta-estimate
> M = sum(rel.w*gstar)
> M

[1] 0.42
```

The variance and CI for the meta-estimate are computed as follows:

```
> # The variance of M
> var.M = 1/tot.w
> var.M

[1] 0.00402

> # The SE
> se.M = sqrt(var.M)
> se.M

[1] 0.0634

> # The lower 95% CI bound
> lowCI.M = M-1.96*se.M
> lowCI.M

[1] 0.296

> # The upper 95% CI bound
> upCI.M = M+1.96*se.M
> upCI.M

[1] 0.544
```

The 95% CI does not cover zero and we conclude that the pooled effect is statistically significant. We calculate the z-value and the associated p-value as follows:

```
> # Compute z
> z = M/se.M
> z

[1] 6.62

> # Compute p-value
> pval  = 2*(1-pnorm(abs(z)))
> pval

[1] 3.54e-11
```

The significant result from this p-value confirms the conclusion from the 95% CI.

For meta-analysis using the random-effects model, we calculate the estimate for τ^2 which is estimated from the Q-statistic as follows:

```
> # The Q statistic
> Q = sum(w*gstar^2)-(sum(w*gstar))^2/tot.w
> Q

[1] 12.3

> # The degrees of freedom from 6 studies
> df= 6-1
> # C quantity
> C = tot.w - sum(w^2)/tot.w
> C

[1] 189

> # The tau-square estimate
> tau2 = (Q-df)/C
> tau2

[1] 0.0383
```

With this estimate, we then calculate the weightings in the random-effects model as follows:

```
> # Now compute the weights incorporating heterogeneity
> wR = 1/(var.gstar+tau2)
> wR

[1] 14.0 14.5 11.3 20.7 12.4 16.2

> # The total weight
> tot.wR = sum(wR)
> tot.wR

[1] 89.1

> # The relative weight
> rel.wR = wR/tot.wR
> rel.wR

[1] 0.157 0.163 0.127 0.232 0.139 0.182
```

Then we calculate the random-effects meta-estimate, its variance and 95% CI as follows:

```
> # The meta-estimate
> MR = sum(rel.wR*gstar)
> MR

[1] 0.359

> # The variance of MR
> var.MR = 1/tot.wR
> var.MR

[1] 0.0112

> # The SE of MR
> se.MR = sqrt(var.MR)
> se.MR

[1] 0.106
```

```
> # The lower bound of 95% CI
> lowCI.MR = MR - 1.96*se.MR
> lowCI.MR

[1] 0.151

> # The upper 95% CI
> upCI.MR = MR + 1.96*se.MR
> upCI.MR

[1] 0.567

> # The z value
> zR = MR/se.MR
> zR

[1] 3.39

> # The p-value
> pval.R = 2*(1-pnorm(abs(zR)))
> pval.R

[1] 0.000703
```

The summary table for the Hedges' estimate and weightings can be printed as:

```
> # The summary table
> sumTab = data.frame(
                SMD          = round(gstar,4),
                lowCI        = round(lowCI.gstar,4),
                upperCI      = round(upCI.gstar,4),
                pctW.fixed   = round(rel.w*100,2),
                pctW.random  = round(rel.wR*100,2))
> rownames(sumTab) = rownames(dat)

> # Print it
> sumTab
```

```
           SMD   lowCI upperCI pctW.fixed pctW.random
Carroll 0.0945 -0.2633   0.452      12.06        15.7
Grant   0.2774 -0.0665   0.621      13.07        16.3
Peck    0.3665 -0.0717   0.805       8.04        12.7
Donat   0.6644  0.4684   0.860      40.21        23.2
Stewart 0.4618  0.0591   0.865       9.52        13.9
Young   0.1852 -0.1155   0.486      17.09        18.2
```

Interested readers should see now that all results from subsection 5.2.3.2 using R library `meta` are reproduced.

5.3 Meta-Analysis of Tubeless vs Standard Percutaneous Nephrolithotomy

As seen from section 5.1.2, the PCNL data is loaded into R from the external Excel file `dat4Meta` and named as `dat` as seen from Table 5.2.

5.3.1 Comparison of Operation Duration

To compare the operation duration for tubeless PCNL and standard PCNL, six of the seven studies were selected for this outcome measure. The authors used mean difference (MD) Δ for their meta-analysis. This analysis can be reproduced using following R code chunk:

```
> # Call metacont for meta analysis
> duration = metacont(n.E,Mean.E, SD.E, n.C, Mean.C, SD.C,
        studlab=Study, data=dat[dat$Outcome=="duration",],
        sm="MD", label.e="Tubeless", label.c="Standard")
> # Print the analysis
> duration
```

```
                        MD          95%-CI  %W(fixed) %W(random)
Ahmet Tefekli 2007   -16.70 [-23.06;-10.337]  16.51   17.7
B.Lojanapiwat 2010    -8.23 [-16.88;  0.422]   8.93   16.0
```

```
Hemendra N. Shah 2008    3.64 [ -2.97; 10.250]  15.30  17.5
Hemendra Shah 2009     -16.00 [-19.97;-12.026]  42.32  19.1
J. Jun-Ou 2010         -11.47 [-18.60; -4.344]  13.16  17.2
Michael Choi 2006        9.14 [ -4.14; 22.418]   3.79  12.5

Number of studies combined: k=6

                          MD           95%-CI      z p.value
Fixed effect model    -10.87  [-13.5; -8.28] -8.24 < 0.0001
Random effects model  -7.51   [-15.2;  0.13] -1.93   0.054

Quantifying heterogeneity:
tau^2 = 75.4491; H = 2.73 [1.92; 3.87]; I^2 = 86.6% [73%; 93.3%]

Test of heterogeneity:
     Q d.f.  p.value
 37.25    5 < 0.0001

Details on meta-analytical method:
- Inverse variance method
- DerSimonian-Laird estimator for tau^2
```

This reproduces all the results. These studies demonstrate statistically significant heterogeneity with $Q = 37.25$ and $d.f. = 5$, which gives a p-value $<$ 0.0001. The authors thus used the random-effects model. From the random-effects model, the estimated MD = -7.51 and the 95% CI is (-15.2, 0.13) which covers zero, indicating a non-statistically significant difference between tubeless PCNL and standard PCNL in terms of operation duration. The z-statistic is -1.93 with p-value of 0.054 again indicating statistical non-significance at the 5% significance level.

Figure 1 in the paper can be reproduced (i.e. Figure 5.2 in this chapter) simply using `forest` from the `meta` package as follows:

```
> forest(duration)
```

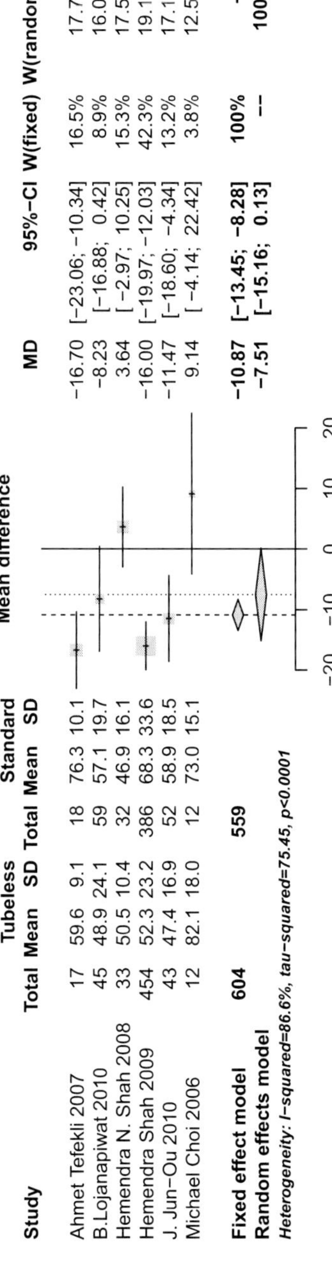

FIGURE 5.2: Forest Plot for Operation Duration

We are compelled to inject a word of caution concerning the conclusion from this meta-analysis. Among the 6 studies, 3 of them (i.e. Ahmet Tefekli 2007, Hemendra Shah 2009, J. Jun-Ou 2010) in fact yielded statistically significant results. In view of this and the fact that the random-effects meta-model yielded a p-value of 0.054 which is marginally statistically insignificant, the weight of evidence does not strongly support lack of a real difference between the two interventions in terms of operation duration. In fact, if the standardized mean difference using Hedges' g is used for meta-analysis, a statistically significant result is revealed as the estimated SMD=-0.410 with 95% CI of (-0.798, -0.0229) and the z-statistic of -2.08 with p-value of 0.0379. The corresponding R code chunk is as follows:

```
> # Call metacont for meta analysis with SMD
> SMD.duration = metacont(n.E,Mean.E, SD.E, n.C, Mean.C, SD.C,
         studlab=Study, data=dat[dat$Outcome=="duration",],
         sm="SMD", label.e="Tubeless", label.c="Standard")
> # Print the analysis
> SMD.duration
```

```
                         SMD            95%-CI  %W(fixed) %W(random)
Ahmet Tefekli 2007    -1.695 [-2.480;-0.9093]   2.25     11.9
B.Lojanapiwat 2010    -0.376 [-0.768; 0.0151]   9.08     18.8
Hemendra N. Shah 2008  0.266 [-0.222; 0.7548]   5.83     17.0
Hemendra Shah 2009    -0.562 [-0.700;-0.4235]  72.66     22.6
J. Jun-Ou 2010        -0.640 [-1.054;-0.2252]   8.09     18.4
Michael Choi 2006      0.532 [-0.285; 1.3487]   2.08     11.4

Number of studies combined: k=6

                         SMD              95%-CI      z  p.value
Fixed effect model   -0.506  [-0.624; -0.3878] -8.41 < 0.0001
Random effects model -0.410  [-0.798; -0.0229] -2.08   0.0379

Quantifying heterogeneity:
tau^2 = 0.1682;H = 2.28[1.56; 3.35]; I^2 = 80.8%[58.7%; 91.1%]
```

```
Test of heterogeneity:
     Q d.f.  p.value
 26.04    5 < 0.0001

 Details on meta-analytical method:
- Inverse variance method
- DerSimonian-Laird estimator for tau^2
```

5.3.2 Comparison of Length of Hospital Stay

To compare the length of hospital stay between tubeless PCNL and tube PCNL, all seven studies are used. The meta-analysis can be performed using the following R code chunk:

```
> LOS = metacont(n.E,Mean.E, SD.E, n.C, Mean.C, SD.C,
                 studlab=Study, data=dat[dat$Outcome=="LOS",],
                 sm="MD", label.e="Tubeless", label.c="Standard")
> # Print the fit
> LOS


                            MD          95%-CI %W(fixed) %W(random)
Ahmet Tefekli 2007      -28.80 [-39.8;-17.828]   1.16      14.20
B.Lojanapiwat 2010      -44.64 [-60.1;-29.164]   0.58      11.50
Hemendra N. Shah 2008    -9.08 [-17.5; -0.691]   1.99      15.74
Hemendra Shah 2009      -22.70 [-29.1;-16.333]   3.45      16.84
J. Jun-Ou 2010          -23.92 [-35.8;-12.057]   0.99      13.65
Madhu S. Agrawal 2008   -32.40 [-33.6;-31.163]  91.44      18.53
Michael Choi 2006        -1.20 [-20.4; 17.993]   0.38       9.54

Number of studies combined: k=7

                          MD           95%-CI     z  p.value
Fixed effect model     -31.4  [-32.6; -30.2] -52.1 < 0.0001
Random effects model -23.9  [-32.4; -15.4]  -5.5 < 0.0001
```

```
Quantifying heterogeneity:
tau^2=101.0369; H =2.91[2.14; 3.97]; I^2=88.2%[78.1%; 93.7%]

Test of heterogeneity:
     Q d.f.  p.value
 50.94    6 < 0.0001

Details on meta-analytical method:
- Inverse variance method
- DerSimonian-Laird estimator for tau^2
```

Similar to the authors, we use the "MD" for this meta-analysis. It can be seen that the test of heterogeneity yields $Q = 50.94$ with $df = 6$ resulting in a p-value < 0.001 from χ^2-test. This indicates statistically significant heterogeneity which leads to the random-effects model. Using the random-effects model, the combined mean difference $MD = -23.86$ hours with 95% of (-32.35,-15.36) which is statistically significant with p-value < 0.0001. This indicated that the mean length of hospital stay for the tubeless PCNL group was statistically significantly shorter than that for standard the PCNL group by a difference of 23.86 hours.

Figure 2 in the paper can be reproduced simply using `forest` from the `meta` package using *forest(LOS)* as seen in Figure 5.3. We note that the results from this analysis matches the results from the authors' Figure 2. We note that there is an obvious typo from the 95% CI reported in the paper as (-39.77,-17.83) which is different from their Figure 2 as well as from the results of our analysis.

The same conclusion may be produced using Hedges' g and we leave this analysis to interested readers.

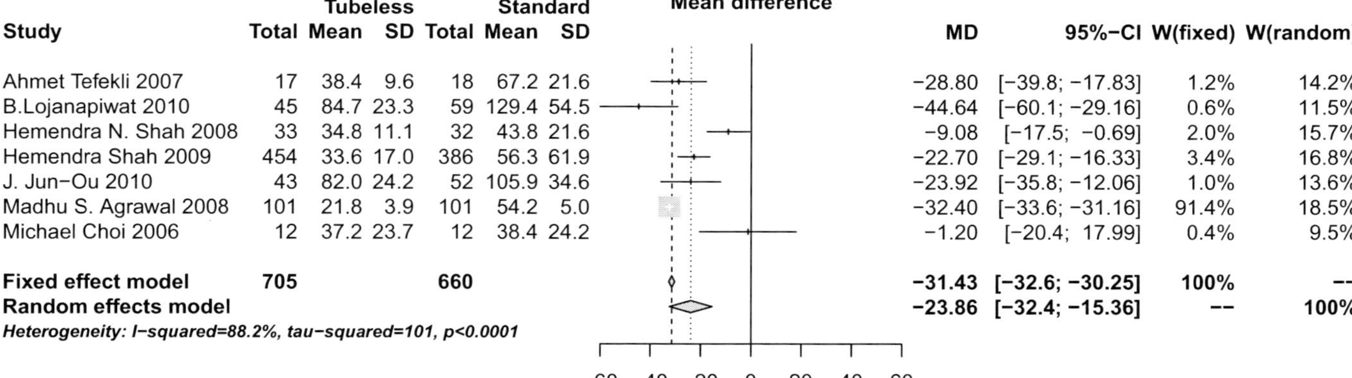

Tubeless
Standard
Mean difference
Study
Total Mean SD Total Mean SD
MD 95%−CI W(fixed) W(random)
Ahmet Tefekli 2007 17 38.4 9.6 18 67.2 21.6 −28.80 [−39.8; −17.83] 1.2% 14.2%
B.Lojanapiwat 2010 45 84.7 23.3 59 129.4 54.5 −44.64 [−60.1; −29.16] 0.6% 11.5%
Hemendra N. Shah 2008 33 34.8 11.1 32 43.8 21.6 −9.08 [−17.5; −0.69] 2.0% 15.7%
Hemendra Shah 2009 454 33.6 17.0 386 56.3 61.9 −22.70 [−29.1; −16.33] 3.4% 16.8%
J. Jun−Ou 2010 43 82.0 24.2 52 105.9 34.6 −23.92 [−35.8; −12.06] 1.0% 13.6%
Madhu S. Agrawal 2008 101 21.8 3.9 101 54.2 5.0 −32.40 [−33.6; −31.16] 91.4% 18.5%
Michael Choi 2006 12 37.2 23.7 12 38.4 24.2 −1.20 [−20.4; 17.99] 0.4% 9.5%
Fixed effect model 705 660 −31.43 [−32.6; −30.25] 100% --
Random effects model −23.86 [−32.4; −15.36] -- 100%
Heterogeneity: I−squared=88.2%, tau−squared=101, p<0.0001
−60 −40 −20 0 20 40 60

FIGURE 5.3: Forest Plot for the Length of Hospital Stay

5.3.3 Comparison of Postoperative Analgesic Requirement

We now compare the tubeless and standard PCNL groups in terms of postoperative analgesic requirement (diclofenac sodium or morphine). As discussed in the paper, the authors selected five of the seven studies for this meta-analysis based on the available data. The meta-analysis is implemented in R with code chunk as follows:

```
> analgesic = metacont(n.E,Mean.E, SD.E, n.C, Mean.C, SD.C,
         studlab=Study, data=dat[dat$Outcome=="analgesic",],
         sm="MD", label.e="Tubeless", label.c="Standard")
> # Print the summary
> analgesic

                           MD          95%-CI  %W(fixed) %W(random)
B.Lojanapiwat 2010      -36.0 [ -49.1; -22.9]   19.18     21.7
Hemendra N. Shah 2008   -96.1 [-162.9; -29.2]    0.74     13.4
Hemendra Shah 2009     -147.2 [-164.1;-130.3]   11.46     21.3
J. Jun-Ou 2010          -33.0 [ -46.5; -19.5]   18.09     21.6
Madhu S. Agrawal 2008   -44.8 [ -52.9; -36.7]   50.53     22.0

Number of studies combined: k=5


                         MD           95%-CI     z  p.value
Fixed effect model    -53.1 [ -58.8;-47.4] -18.2 < 0.0001
Random effects model -69.0 [-107.7;-30.4]   -3.5   0.0005

Quantifying heterogeneity:
tau^2 = 1749.7704; H = 5.9 [4.61; 7.56]; I^2 = 97.1% [95.3%; 98.3%]

Test of heterogeneity:
      Q d.f.  p.value
 139.45    4 < 0.0001

Details on meta-analytical method:
- Inverse variance method
- DerSimonian-Laird estimator for tau^2
```

We note from the analysis that the test of heterogeneity is statistically significant with p-value < 0.0001 ($Q = 139.45$, df $= 4$) and the random-effects model showed that the mean analgesic requirement for the tubeless PCNL was statistically significantly lower than that from the standard PCNL with a combined mean difference of 69.02 mg, postoperative analgesic requirement p-value < 0.05 and associated 95% CI of (-107.67, -30.36).

Interested readers are encouraged to reproduce the `forest` plot for this analysis as well as the meta-analysis using Hedges g for standardized mean difference modifying the corresponding R code.

5.3.4 Comparison of Postoperative Haematocrit Change

To compare the two PCNL groups in terms of postoperative hematocrit changes, the authors selected four of the seven studies based on the available data for their meta-analysis using the "MD". The implementation in R is as follows:

```
> haematocrit = metacont(n.E,Mean.E, SD.E, n.C, Mean.C, SD.C,
        studlab=Study,data=dat[dat$Outcome=="haematocrit",],
        sm="MD", label.e="Tubeless", label.c="Standard")
> # Print the summary
> haematocrit

                         MD          95%-CI %W(fixed) %W(random)
Ahmet Tefekli 2007     0.40 [ 0.1002;0.6998]  2.09    18.5
Hemendra N. Shah 2008 -0.06 [-0.4658;0.3458]  1.14    12.7
Hemendra Shah 2009    -0.15 [-0.3281;0.0281]  5.93    28.7
Madhu S. Agrawal 2008 -0.03 [-0.0755;0.0155] 90.84    40.1

Number of studies combined: k=4

                          MD            95%-CI      z  p.value
Fixed effect model   -0.0285 [-0.0718;0.0149] -1.286 0.1984
Random effects model  0.0113 [-0.1625;0.1851]  0.127 0.8988

Quantifying heterogeneity:
```

```
tau^2=0.0191;H=1.79[1.06;3.05];I^2=68.9%[10.3%;89.3%]

Test of heterogeneity:
    Q d.f.  p.value
 9.66    3   0.0217

Details on meta-analytical method:
- Inverse variance method
- DerSimonian-Laird estimator for tau^2
```

From the analysis, there is statistically significant heterogeneity among the 4 studies with p-value $= 0.0217$ ($Q = 9.66$, df $= 3$). With the random-effects model, the results showed that the difference in the hematocrit change between the tubeless group and the standard PCNL group was not statistically significant (p-value $= 0.8988$); the combined mean difference $MD = 0.0113$ with a 95% CI of (-0.1625, 0.1851).

5.3.5 Conclusions and Discussion

We re-analyzed the data from Wang et al. (2011) to compare tubeless vs standard percutaneous nephrolithotomy (PCNL) using the R package `meta` and reproduced the results from the paper. This analysis demonstrated that tubeless PCNL is a good option to standard PCNL with the advantages of significantly reduced hospital stay and less need for postoperative analgesia. The analysis also showed that there was no significant difference between the groups in terms of haematocrit change after surgery. The authors concluded that there was no difference in operation duration based on the mean difference with a very marginally statistically insignificant p-value of 0.054. We re-analyzed the data using the Hedges' g using the standardized mean difference and revealed a statistically significant difference of -0.4104 with p-value of 0.0379.

5.4 Discussion

In this chapter, we illustrated meta-analysis methods for endpoints or summary statistics of continuous data arising in clinical trials and other studies. Two commonly used methods were described based on synthesizing the mean difference and Hedges' standardized mean difference g. Two datasets were used to show detailed step-by-step implementation of these methods.

The first dataset reflecting the impact of some intervention on reading scores in children from Borenstein et al. (2009) was used to illustrate the methods with step-by-step implementation in R in comparison with the R package `meta` so that readers may understand the methods in depth. The second dataset from Wang et al. (2011) provided endpoints reflecting a set of 7 studies that compared the effects of tubeless vs standard percutaneous nephrolithotomy on several continuous measures. We illustrated meta-analyses of this dataset using the R package `meta` to reproduce the results from this paper.

Chapter 6

Heterogeneity in Meta-Analysis

So far we have illustrated all the concepts in the output from meta-analysis using R except heterogeneity measures. Discerning readers may have noticed that whenever we called `metabin` or `metacont` from R package `meta` for meta-analysis as seen in Chapters 4 and 5, two other items appeared in the output as `Quantifying heterogeneity` and `Test of heterogeneity`. These heterogeneity measures are discussed in this chapter.

In Section 3.2.3 for the random-effects meta-analysis model, we introduced a quantity Q to be used to estimate the between-study variance τ^2; i.e. Q is a measure of heterogeneity. In this chapter, we discuss this measure of heterogeneity, used for `Test of heterogeneity` in Section 6.1 along with other heterogeneity measures τ^2, H and I^2 from R output `Quantifying heterogeneity` in Section 6.2. The step-by-step implementation will be illustrated in Section 6.3. Discussion appears in Section 6.4.

6.1 Heterogeneity Quantity Q and the `Test of heterogeneity` in R `meta`

Introduced in Section 3.2.3, Q is used to quantify the heterogeneity across all studies and included both the true effect sizes and the random errors from the random-effects model of (3.11). As seen in Section 3.2.3, Q is defined as follows:

$$Q = \sum_{i=1}^{K} w_i(\hat{\delta}_i - \hat{\delta})^2 \qquad (6.1)$$

where w_i is the weight from the ith study, $\hat{\delta}_i$ is the ith study effect size, and $\hat{\delta}$ is the summary effect. It can be seen that Q is calculated as: 1) compute the deviations of each effect size from the meta-estimate and square them (i.e. $(\hat{\delta}_i - \hat{\delta})^2$), 2) weight these values by the inverse-variance for each study, and 3) then sum these values across all K studies to produce a weighted sum of squares (WSS) to obtain the heterogeneity measure Q.

From equation (3.25), we have shown that the expected value of Q (i.e. (DerSimonian and Laird, 1986)) is:

$$E(Q) = (K-1) + \tau^2 \left[\sum_{i=1}^{K} w_i - \frac{\sum_{i=1}^{K} w_i^2}{\sum_{i=1}^{K} w_i} \right] \tag{6.2}$$

Under the assumption of no heterogeneity (all studies have the same effect size), then τ^2 would be zero and $E(Q) = df = K - 1$.

Based on this heterogeneity measure Q, the `Test of heterogeneity` is conducted and addresses the null hypothesis that the effect sizes δ_i from all studies share a common effect size δ (i.e. the assumption of homogeneity) and then test this hypothesis where the test statistic is constructed using Q as a central χ^2 distribution with degrees of freedom of $df = K - 1$ as defined by Cochran (1952) and Cochran (1954). Under this testing procedure, the associated p-value for the calculated Q is reported in the R output to test for the existence of heterogeneity. The typical significance level for this test is α at 0.05. If the p-value is less than α we reject the null hypothesis and conclude heterogeneity, that all the studies do not share a common effect size.

The reader should be cautioned that there is a disadvantage of the χ^2-test using the Q-statistic; i.e. it has poor statistical power to detect true heterogeneity for a meta-analysis with a small number of studies, but excessive power to detect negligible variability with a large number of studies - as discussed in Harwell (1997) and Hardy and Thompson (1998). Thus, a nonsignificant Q-test from a small number of studies can lead to an erroneous selection of a fixed-effects model when there is possible true heterogeneity among the studies, and vice versa. The inability to conclude statistically significant heterogeneity in a meta-analysis of a small number of studies at the 0.05 level of significance is similar to failing to detect statistically significant treatment-by-center interaction in a multicenter clinical trial. In these settings, many analysts will conduct the test of homogeneity at the 0.10 level, as a means of increasing power of the test.

6.2 The *Quantifying Heterogeneity* in R `meta`

We used the Q-statistic to test the existence of heterogeneity in the above section and report the p-value for the test. However, this test only informs us about the presence versus the absence of heterogeneity, but it does not report the extent of such heterogeneity. We will discuss other measures of the "extent" and magnitude of this heterogeneity using the Q-statistic and quantify heterogeneity of the true dispersion among the studies. As seen from the R output, several heterogeneity indices: τ^2, H and I^2, are commonly used to describe and report the magnitude of the dispersion of true effect sizes.

6.2.1 The τ^2 Index

The τ^2 index is defined as the variance of the true effect sizes as seen in the random-effects model (3.11). Since it is impossible to observe the true effect sizes, we cannot calculate this variance directly, but we can estimate it from the observed data using equation (6.1) as follows:

$$\hat{\tau}^2 = \frac{Q - (K-1)}{U} \tag{6.3}$$

which is the well-known DerSimonian-Laird method of moments for τ^2 in equation (3.18). Even though the true variance τ^2 can never be less than zero, the estimated variance $\hat{\tau}^2$ can sometimes be from the sampling error leading to $Q < K - 1$. When this occurs, the estimated $\hat{\tau}^2$ is set to zero.

As used in the random-effects model, the τ^2 index is also an estimate for the between-studies variance in the meta-analysis of the true effects.

6.2.2 The H Index

Another index or measure of heterogeneity is the H, proposed in Higgins and Thompson (2002), and defined as follows:

$$H = \sqrt{\frac{Q}{K-1}} \tag{6.4}$$

This index is based on the fact that $E[Q] = K - 1$ when there is no heterogeneity. In this case, H should be 1.

The confidence interval for the H index is derived in Higgins and Thompson (2002) based on the assumption that the natural logarithm of $\ln(H)$ follows a standard normal distribution. Accordingly:

$$LL_H = \exp\left\{\ln(H) - |z_{\alpha/2}| \times SE\left[\ln(H)\right]\right\} \tag{6.5}$$

$$UL_H = \exp\left\{\ln(H) + |z_{\alpha/2}| \times SE\left[\ln(H)\right]\right\} \tag{6.6}$$

where LL and UL denote the lower- and upper-limits of the CI, $z_{\alpha/2}$ is the $\alpha/2$-quantile of the standard normal distribution, and $SE[\ln(H)]$ is the standard error of $\ln(H)$ and is estimated by

$$SE\left[\ln(H)\right] = \begin{cases} \frac{1}{2}\frac{\ln(Q)-\ln(K-1)}{\sqrt{2Q-\sqrt{2K-3}}} & \text{if } Q > K \\ \sqrt{\frac{1}{2(K-2)}\left(1-\frac{1}{3(K-2)^2}\right)} & \text{if } Q \leq K \end{cases} \tag{6.7}$$

Since $E(Q) \approx K - 1$ as seen equation (6.2), the H index should be greater than 1 to measure the relative magnitude of heterogeneity among all the studies. If the lower limit of this interval is greater than 1, the H is statistically significant and the `Test of heterogeneity` should be significant also.

6.2.3 The I^2 Index

To measure the proportion of observed heterogeneity from the real heterogeneity, Higgins and Thompson (2002) and Higgins et al. (2003) proposed the I^2 index as follows:

$$I^2 = \left(\frac{Q-(K-1)}{Q}\right) \times 100\%, \tag{6.8}$$

which again represents the ratio of excess dispersion to total dispersion and is similar to the well-known R^2 in classical regression which represents the proportion of the total variance that can be explained by the regression variables.

As suggested from Higgins et al. (2003) a value of the I^2 index around 25%, 50%, and 75% could be considered as *low-*, *moderate-*, and *high*-heterogeneity, respectively. As noted in their paper, about half of the meta-analyses of clinical trials in the *Cochrane Database of Systematic Reviews* reported an I^2 index of zero and the rest reported evenly distributed I^2 indices between 0% and 100%.

Mathematically, the I^2 index can be represented using the H index as follows:

$$I^2 = \frac{H^2 - 1}{H^2} \times 100\% \tag{6.9}$$

This expression allows us to use the results from the H index to give a confidence interval for the I^2 index using the expressions in equations (6.5) and (6.6) as follows:

$$\begin{aligned} LL_{I^2} &= \left[\frac{(LL_H)^2 - 1}{(LL_H)^2}\right] \times 100\% \\ UL_{I^2} &= \left[\frac{(UL_H)^2 - 1}{(UL_H)^2}\right] \times 100\% \end{aligned}$$

Since I^2 represents the percentage, any of these limits which is computed as negative is set to zero. In the case that the lower limit of I^2 is greater than zero, then the I^2 is regarded as statistically significant and the `Test of heterogeneity` should be significant also.

6.3 Step-By-Step Implementations in R

We illustrate the implementation in R re-using the Cochrane Collaboration Logo data from Chapter 3 and the tubeless vs standard PCNL data from Chapter 5.

6.3.1 Cochrane Collaboration Logo Data

The data from Table 3.1 can be accessed from the R library `rmeta` and is named `dat` for easy reference.

This is a binary data set and we only illustrate the step-by-step implementation in R for the risk-ratio(RR). The computations using the risk difference and odds-ratio can be easily done following the code in this chapter and is left for interested readers as practice.

6.3.1.1 Illustration Using R Library meta

For comparison, we first output the results using the R library in this subsection as reference for the next subsection in R step-by-step implementation.

The implementation in the R library meta can be easily done using the following R code chunk:

```
> # Risk-ratio using "inverse weighting"
> RR.Cochrane = metabin(ev.trt,n.trt,ev.ctrl,n.ctrl,studlab=name,
                 data=dat, method="Inverse", sm="RR")
> # Print the result
> RR.Cochrane

                RR             95%-CI %W(fixed) %W(random)
Auckland     0.607  [0.4086; 0.901]     53.02      42.19
Block        0.177  [0.0212; 1.472]      1.85       2.65
Doran        0.283  [0.0945; 0.846]      6.90       9.18
Gamsu        0.732  [0.3862; 1.388]     20.26      22.56
Morrison     0.377  [0.1022; 1.394]      4.86       6.66
Papageorgiou 0.151  [0.0190; 1.196]      1.93       2.77
Tauesch      1.014  [0.4287; 2.400]     11.18      13.99

Number of studies combined: k=7

                        RR            95%-CI     z  p.value
Fixed effect model   0.589  [0.442; 0.785] -3.60   0.0003
Random effects model 0.572  [0.403; 0.812] -3.13   0.0018

Quantifying heterogeneity:
tau^2 = 0.0349; H = 1.09 [1; 1.56]; I^2 = 15.1% [0%; 58.8%]

Test of heterogeneity:
```

```
    Q d.f. p.value
 7.06    6   0.315

Details on meta-analytical method:
- Inverse variance method
- DerSimonian-Laird estimator for tau^2
```

From the output, we see that the risk-ratio from the fixed-effects model is RR = 0.589 with 95% CI of (0.442, 0.785) and the value of the z-statistic is -3.60 with a p-value of 0.0003; whereas the risk-ratio from the random-effects model is RR=0.572 with 95% CI of (0.403, 0.812) and the value of the z-statistic is -3.13 with a p-value of 0.0018. This again indicates that there was a significant overall effect for steroid treatment in reducing neonatal death.

For `Test of heterogeneity`, the Q-statistic = 7.06 with df = 6 which yields a p-value from the χ^2 distribution of 0.315, indicating there is no statistically significant heterogeneity among the 7 studies. From `Quantifying heterogeneity`, the estimated between-study variance is $\tau^2 = 0.0349$, which is very small; the H index is 1.09 with 95% CI of (1, 1.56) with lower limit of 1, which indicates insignificant heterogeneity. Finally $I^2 = 15.1\%$ with 95% CI of (0%, 58.8%) where the lower limit of 0 again indicates insignificant heterogeneity.

6.3.1.2 Implementation in R: Step-by-Step

To calculate the risk-ratio using R we proceed as follows:

```
> # Calculate the risks from the treatment group
> pE = dat$ev.trt/dat$n.trt
> pE

[1] 0.0677 0.0145 0.0494 0.1069 0.0448 0.0141 0.1429

> # Calculate the risks from the control group
> pC = dat$ev.ctrl/dat$n.ctrl
> pC

[1] 0.1115 0.0820 0.1746 0.1460 0.1186 0.0933 0.1408
```

```
> # Then calculate the risk-ratio as effect size
> ES = pE/pC
> ES

[1] 0.607 0.177 0.283 0.732 0.377 0.151 1.014
```

For the risk-ratio, it is common practice to use its natural logarithm to calculate the confidence interval (CI) and then transform back to get the CI for the RR. This process can be implemented as follows:

```
> # Calculate the log risk ratio
> lnES = log(ES)
> lnES

[1] -0.4996 -1.7327 -1.2629 -0.3119 -0.9745 -1.8911
[7]  0.0142

> # Calculate the variance of the logged RR
> VlnES =1/dat$ev.trt-1/dat$n.trt+1/dat$ev.ctrl-1/dat$n.ctrl
> VlnES

[1] 0.0407 1.1691 0.3127 0.1065 0.4443 1.1154 0.1931

> # Then the upper CI limit
> ciup   = lnES+1.96*sqrt(VlnES)
> ciup

[1] -0.104  0.387 -0.167  0.328  0.332  0.179  0.875

> # The lower CI limit
> cilow   = lnES-1.96*sqrt(VlnES)
> cilow

[1] -0.895 -3.852 -2.359 -0.952 -2.281 -3.961 -0.847

> # Then transform back to the original scale
> cat("The low CI is:", exp(cilow),"\n\n")

The low CI is: 0.409 0.0212 0.0945 0.386 0.102 0.019 0.429
```

```
> cat("The upper CI is:", exp(ciup),"\n\n")

The upper CI is: 0.901 1.47 0.846 1.39 1.39 1.2 2.4
```

This reproduces the summary statistics from the R output in subsection 6.3.1.1. We now calculate the statistics from the fixed-effects model as follows:

```
> # The inverse of variance for each study
> fwi      = 1/VlnES
> fwi

[1] 24.566  0.855  3.198  9.390  2.251  0.897  5.180

> # The total weight
> fw       = sum(fwi)
> fw

[1] 46.3

> # The relative weight for each study
> rw       = fwi/fw
> rw

[1] 0.5302 0.0185 0.0690 0.2026 0.0486 0.0193 0.1118

> # The fixed-effects weighted mean estimate
> flnES    = sum(lnES*rw)
> flnES

[1] -0.53

> # The variance for the weighted mean
> var      = 1/fw
> var

[1] 0.0216

> # Then the fixed-effects meta-estimate of RR
> fRR      = exp(flnES)
> fRR
```

```
[1] 0.589

> # The lower limit
> fLL     = exp(flnES-1.96*sqrt(var))
> fLL

[1] 0.442

> # The upper limit
> fUL     = exp(flnES+1.96*sqrt(var))
> fUL

[1] 0.785
```

Again this reproduces the weightings and the meta-estimate from the fixed-effects model in the R output in subsection 6.3.1.1. The statistics from the random-effects model can be calculated as follows:

```
> # Calculate the Q-statistic
> Q       = sum(fwi*lnES^2)-(sum(fwi*lnES))^2/fw
> Q

[1] 7.06

> # The number of studies and df
> K       = dim(dat)[1]
> df      = K -1
> # The U-statistic
> U       = fw - sum(fwi^2)/fw
> U

[1] 30.5

> # Then the estimate tau-square
> tau2    = ifelse(Q > K-1,(Q-df)/U,0)
> tau2

[1] 0.0349
```

This reproduces the between-study variance of $\hat{\tau}^2$=0.0349. With this estimate of τ^2, we can reproduce the statistics from random-effects model as follows:

```
> # Compute the weights from random-effects model
> wR      = 1/(VlnES+tau2)
> wR

[1] 13.223  0.831  2.877  7.071  2.087  0.869  4.386

> # The total weight
> tot.wR = sum(wR)
> # The relative weight
> rel.wR = wR/tot.wR
> rel.wR

[1] 0.4219 0.0265 0.0918 0.2256 0.0666 0.0277 0.1399

> # Then the weighted mean from random-effects model
> rlnES = sum(lnES*rel.wR)
> rlnES

[1] -0.558

> # The variance for the weighted mean
> var    = 1/tot.wR
> var

[1] 0.0319

> # Transform back to the original scale
> rRR    =  exp(rlnES)
> rRR

[1] 0.572

> # The lower limits
> rLL    = exp(rlnES-1.96*sqrt(var))
> rLL
```

```
[1] 0.403

> # The upper limits
> rUL    = exp(rlnES+1.96*sqrt(var))
> rUL

[1] 0.812

> # The z-statistic
> zR     = rlnES/sqrt(var)
> zR

[1] -3.13

> # The p-value
> pval.R = 2*(1-pnorm(abs(zR)))
> pval.R

[1] 0.00177
```

This reproduces the weightings and the meta-estimate from the random-effects model in the R output in subsection 6.3.1.1.

Now we consider the measures of heterogeneity. For `Test of heterogeneity`, we found that $Q = 7.0638$ with df=6 above. The associated p-value can be then calculated as follows:

```
> pval4Q =  pchisq(Q, df, lower.tail=F)
> pval4Q

[1] 0.315
```

which indicates that there is no statistically significant heterogeneity. We found the estimate of $\hat{\tau}^2$=0.0349 above. The H index and its 95% CI can be calculated as follows:

```
> # The H index
> H = sqrt(Q/df)
> H

[1] 1.09
```

```
> # The SE for logH
> se.logH=ifelse(Q>K,0.5*(log(Q)-log(K-1))/(sqrt(2*Q)-sqrt(2*K-3)),
                 sqrt(1/(2*(K-2))*(1-1/(3*(K-2)^2))))
> se.logH

[1] 0.185

> # The lower limit
> LL.H  = max(1,exp(log(H) -1.96*se.logH))
> LL.H

[1] 1

> # The upper limit
> UL.H  = exp(log(H) +1.96*se.logH)
> UL.H

[1] 1.56
```

The I^2 index and its 95% CI are then calculated as follows:

```
> # The I-square
> I2 = (Q-df)/Q*100
> I2

[1] 15.1

> # The lower limit for I-square
> LL.I2 = max(0,(LL.H^2-1)/LL.H^2*100)
> LL.I2

[1] 0

> # The upper limit for I-square
> UL.I2 = max(0,(UL.H^2-1)/UL.H^2*100)
> UL.I2

[1] 58.8
```

This reproduces all the measures from `Quantifying heterogeneity` from R library `meta` in subsection 6.3.1.1.

6.3.2 Tubeless vs Standard PCNL Data

In Chapter 5, we made use of the meta-analysis from Wang et al. (2011) on tubeless percutaneous nephrolithotomy (PCNL) with standard PCNL for stones of the kidney or upper ureter. In this paper, several outcome measures were used including the operation duration, length of hospital stay, analgesic requirement after tubeless PCNL and pre- and postoperative hematocrit changes. We reproduced all the results in this paper using R in Section 5.3 except finding a slightly different conclusion in operation duration in Subsection 5.3.1 if the analysis is performed using the standardized mean difference (i.e. SMD).

In this section, we use this analysis to illustrate the presentation of heterogeneity for continuous data. As seen from section 5.3, the PCNL data is loaded into R from the external excel file dat4Meta and named as dat for R implementation. To reuse the data and R code, we subset the duration data and again name this subset as dat for analysis in this subsection and those that follow.

6.3.2.1 Implementation in R Library meta

For comparison, we first output the results using the R library in this subsection as reference for the next subsection in R step-by-step implementation. The implementation in the R library meta can be done easily using the following R code chunk:

```
> # Call "metacont" for meta-analysis
> SMD.duration = metacont(n.E,Mean.E, SD.E, n.C, Mean.C, SD.C,
                 studlab=Study, data=dat, sm="SMD",
                 label.e="Tubeless", label.c="Standard")
> # Print the summary
> SMD.duration
```

```
                           SMD            95%-CI %W(fixed) %W(random)
Ahmet Tefekli 2007      -1.695 [-2.480;-0.9093]     2.25     11.9
B.Lojanapiwat 2010      -0.376 [-0.768; 0.0151]     9.08     18.8
Hemendra N. Shah 2008    0.266 [-0.222; 0.7548]     5.83     17.0
Hemendra Shah 2009      -0.562 [-0.700;-0.4235]    72.66     22.6
```

```
J. Jun-Ou 2010        -0.640 [-1.054;-0.2252]   8.09   18.4
Michael Choi 2006      0.532 [-0.285; 1.3487]   2.08   11.4

Number of studies combined: k=6

                          SMD           95%-CI     z    p.value
Fixed effect model     -0.506 [-0.624;-0.3878] -8.41 < 0.0001
Random effects model -0.410 [-0.798;-0.0229] -2.08   0.0379

Quantifying heterogeneity:
tau^2=0.1682; H=2.28[1.56;3.35]; I^2=80.8%[58.7%; 91.1%]

Test of heterogeneity:
     Q d.f.  p.value
 26.04    5 < 0.0001

Details on meta-analytical method:
- Inverse variance method
- DerSimonian-Laird estimator for tau^2
```

From this output, we can see that the `Test of heterogeneity` has a Q-statistic value of 26.04 with $df = 5$ and a p-value < 0.0001, indicating statistically significant heterogeneity among the 6 studies. The measures of heterogeneity in `Quantifying heterogeneity` are $\tau^2 = 0.1682$, $H = 2.28$ with 95% CI (1.56, 3.35) and $I^2 = 80.8\%$ with 95% CI (58.7%, 91.1%), respectively. From the CIs of H and I^2, we can also conclude the existence of statistically significant heterogeneity.

From the fixed-effects model, the standardized mean difference from all 6 studies is SMD=-0.506 with 95% CI of (-0.624, -0.388), the estimated $\hat{\tau}^2$=0.1682, and the estimated SMD = -0.410 with 95% CI of (-0.798, -0.0229) - which are statistically significant.

6.3.2.2 Implementation in R: Step-by-Step

To be consistent with the notation used in the R library `meta` we rename the variables as follows:

```
> dat$n.t = dat$n.E
> dat$n.c = dat$n.C
> dat$m.t = dat$Mean.E
> dat$m.c = dat$Mean.C
> dat$sd.t = dat$SD.E
> dat$sd.c = dat$SD.C
```

Then we calculate the pooled standard deviation as follows:

```
> # Get the pooled sd to calculate the SMD
> pooled.sd = sqrt(((dat$n.t-1)*dat$sd.t^2+
        (dat$n.c-1)*dat$sd.c^2)/(dat$n.t+dat$n.c-2))
> pooled.sd

[1]  9.63 21.71 13.51 28.45 17.79 16.59
```

With the pooled SD, we then calculate Hedges' standardized mean difference (SMD) with correction for unbiased estimate as follows:

```
> # Calculate the standardized mean difference(SMD)
> g = (dat$m.t-dat$m.c)/pooled.sd
> g

[1] -1.735 -0.379  0.269 -0.562 -0.645  0.551

> # Hedges' correction factor
> N = dat$n.t+dat$n.c
> J = 1- 3/(4*N-9)
> J

[1] 0.977 0.993 0.988 0.999 0.992 0.966

> # Now the Hedges' gstar
> gstar = J*g
> gstar

[1] -1.695 -0.376  0.266 -0.562 -0.640  0.532
```

We compute the variance of this SMD as follows:

```
> # Calculate the variance of Hedges's SMD
> var.gstar = (dat$n.t+dat$n.c)/(dat$n.t*dat$n.c) +
                gstar^2/(2*(dat$n.t+dat$n.c-3.94))
> var.gstar

[1] 0.16062 0.03988 0.06213 0.00498 0.04473 0.17372
```

Therefore the 95% CI for all 6 studies can be constructed as:

```
> # The lower limit
> lowCI.gstar = gstar-1.96*sqrt(var.gstar)
> lowCI.gstar

[1] -2.480 -0.768 -0.222 -0.700 -1.054 -0.285

> # The upper limit
> upCI.gstar = gstar+1.96*sqrt(var.gstar)
> upCI.gstar

[1] -0.9093  0.0151  0.7548 -0.4235 -0.2252  1.3487
```

The above calculations reproduce the summary statistics from Section 6.3.2.1. For the fixed-effects model, we first calculate the weights using following R code chunk:

```
> # Calculate the individual weight
> w = 1/var.gstar
> w

[1]   6.23  25.08  16.09 200.72  22.35   5.76

> # The total weight
> tot.w = sum(w)
> tot.w

[1] 276

> # Then the relative weight
> rel.w = w/tot.w
> rel.w
```

```
[1] 0.0225 0.0908 0.0583 0.7266 0.0809 0.0208
```

With these weights, we calculate the meta-estimate as:

```
> # The meta-estimate
> M = sum(rel.w*g)
> M

[1] -0.507
```

Then the variance, and CI computed as:

```
> # The variance of M
> var.M = 1/tot.w
> var.M

[1] 0.00362

> # The SE
> se.M = sqrt(var.M)
> se.M

[1] 0.0602

> # The 95% CI
> lowCI.M = M-1.96*se.M
> lowCI.M

[1] -0.625

> upCI.M = M+1.96*se.M
> upCI.M

[1] -0.389
```

The 95% CI does not cover zero and we conclude that the pooled effect is statistically significant. We can also calculate the z-value and the associated p-value as follows:

```
> # compute z
> z = M/se.M
> z
```

```
[1] -8.43

> # compute p-value
> pval = 2*(1-pnorm(abs(z)))
> pval

[1] 0
```

Again this reproduces the summary statistics from Section 6.3.2.1. For the random-effects model, we calculate the estimate of between-study variance τ^2 which is estimated from the Q-statistic as follows:

```
> # Calculate the heterogeneity Q statistic
> Q  = sum(w*gstar^2)-(sum(w*gstar))^2/tot.w
> Q

[1] 26

> # The number of studies
> K  =6
> # The degrees of freedom
> df = K-1
> # The U quantity
> U  = tot.w - sum(w^2)/tot.w
> U

[1] 125

> # Now we can calculate the tau-square estimate
> tau2 = (Q-df)/U
> tau2

[1] 0.168
```

With this estimate, we can then calculate the weightings in the random-effects model as follows:

```
> # Compute the weights in the random-effects model
> wR = 1/(var.gstar+tau2)
> wR
```

```
[1] 3.04 4.81 4.34 5.77 4.70 2.92

> # The total weight
> tot.wR = sum(wR)
> tot.wR

[1] 25.6

> # The relative weight
> rel.wR = wR/tot.wR
> rel.wR

[1] 0.119 0.188 0.170 0.226 0.184 0.114
```

Then we calculate the meta-estimate, its variance and 95% CI as follows:

```
> # The meta-estimate from the random-effects model
> MR = sum(rel.wR*gstar)
> MR

[1] -0.41

> # The var and SE of MR
> var.MR = 1/tot.wR
> var.MR

[1] 0.0391

> se.MR = sqrt(var.MR)
> se.MR

[1] 0.198

> # The 95% CI
> lowCI.MR = MR - 1.96*se.MR
> lowCI.MR

[1] -0.798

> upCI.MR = MR + 1.96*se.MR
> upCI.MR
```

```
[1] -0.0229
```

```
> # The z value
> zR = MR/se.MR
> zR
```

```
[1] -2.08
```

```
> # The p-value
> pval.R = 2*(1-pnorm(abs(zR)))
> pval.R
```

```
[1] 0.0379
```

These calculations reproduce the summary statistics for both fixed-effect and random-effect models from Section 6.3.2.1.

We now consider the `Test of heterogeneity`. We know that the Q-statistic is:

```
> Q
```

```
[1] 26
```

With $df = K - 1$=6-1=5, the p-value can be calculated as:

```
> pval.HG = 1-pchisq(Q,df)
> pval.HG
```

```
[1] 8.75e-05
```

which is less than 0.05, and we reject the null hypothesis that all studies share a common effect size and conclude that the true effect is not the same in all studies. With this conclusion, we compute other heterogeneity indices in `Quantifying heterogeneity` as follows:

```
> # Calculate the H index
> H = sqrt(Q/df)
> H
```

```
[1] 2.28
```

```
> # The standard error of log(H)
> se.logH = ifelse(Q > K, 0.5*((log(Q)-log(K-1))
                 /(sqrt(2*Q)-sqrt(2*K-3)),
                 sqrt(1/(2*(K-2))*(1-1/(3*(k-2)^2))))
> se.logH

[1] 0.196

> # The lower limit of 95% CI
> LL.H = max(1,exp(log(H) -1.96*se.logH))
> LL.H

[1] 1.56

> # The upper limit of 95% CI
> UL.H  = exp(log(H) +1.96*se.logH)
> UL.H

[1] 3.35

> # Calculate the heterogeneity I-square index
> I2 = (Q-df)/Q*100
> I2

[1] 80.8

> # The lower limit of I-square index
> LL.I2 = max(0,(LL.H^2-1)/LL.H^2*100)
> LL.I2

[1] 58.7

> # The upper limit of I-square index
> UL.I2 = max(0,(UL.H^2-1)/UL.H^2*100)
> UL.I2

[1] 91.1
```

Again these calculations reproduce the summary statistics for heterogeneity from Section 6.3.2.1.

6.4 Discussion

In this chapter, we discussed and illustrated measures of heterogeneity used in meta-analysis. The test of heterogeneity is based on the quantity Q which is distributed as a χ^2 with degrees of freedom of $K-1$. Three other heterogeneity indices were discussed. These are τ^2 to estimate the between-study variance and to be incorporated into random-effect model, H to estimate a standardized heterogeneity index on Q, and I^2 to estimate the proportion of true dispersion from the total dispersion.

The step-by-step implementation in R was illustrated using two datasets. This illustration should help readers understand the methods when they perform their own meta-analyses.

We did not specifically provide detailed calculations for the 95% CI of τ^2 and τ in this chapter. The CI can be easily obtained from the relationship between τ^2 and the H index. From equation (6.3), we obtain

$$\hat{\tau}^2 = \frac{df\left(H^2-1\right)}{U} \tag{6.10}$$

Then the CI limits for H from equations (6.5) and (6.6) can be used to construct the CI for τ^2 as follows:

$$\begin{aligned} LL_{\tau^2} &= \frac{df\left(LL_H^2-1\right)}{U} \\ UL_{\tau^2} &= \frac{df\left(UL_H^2-1\right)}{U} \end{aligned}$$

and consequently the 95% CI for τ can be constructed as follows:

$$\begin{aligned} LL_{\tau} &= \sqrt{LL_{\tau^2}} \\ UL_{\tau} &= \sqrt{UL_{\tau^2}}. \end{aligned}$$

We have concentrated our attention to reproducing the output from R. Interested readers can refer to Bohning et al. (2002) for a more general discussion in estimating heterogeneity with the DerSimonian-Laird estimator. This estimator is commonly used in meta-analysis. More detailed derivation of these heterogeneity indices can be found from Higgins and Thompson (2002).

We indicated in Section 3.4 of Chapter 3 that the choice between a fixed-effects model or random-effects model should not be based on a test of heterogeneity. Rather the choice should be based on a detailed inspection of all aspects of the individual studies that we desire synthesizing the treatment effects. Following this review if it is reasonable to believe 'a priori' that each study would provide an estimate of the same (or common) treatment effect, then a fixed-effects model should be used. Otherwise, use a random-effects model. Further we noted that in practice both models are usually used and the results reported.

So the practical utility of the methods presented in this chapter to assess heterogeneity is to additionally inform the consumer of the meta-analytic results. Following the presentation of synthesized results from a random-effects model, the assessment of heterogeneity using methods described in this chapter would be presented. The consumer would then know the extent to which differences in the observed treatment effects among individual studies was due not only to within study sampling error but also due to between study variability as well - as pointed out in Hedges and Vevea (1998) and Field (2003).

Another way to deal with between-study heterogeneity is to link the heterogeneity with other moderators such as meta-regression which is the focus of the next chapter.

Chapter 7

Meta-Regression

Continuing from Chapter 6 to explain heterogeneity in meta-analysis, we explore meta-regression in this chapter to explain extra heterogeneity (or the residual heterogeneity) using study-level moderators or study-level independent variables. With study-level moderators associated with the reported effect sizes as the dependent variable and their variance as weights, typical weighted regression analysis methods can be utilized. From this point of view, meta-regression is merely typical multiple regression applied for study-level data and therefore the theory of regression can be directly applied for meta-regression.

From the practical side, meta-regression can be used to determine whether continuous or discrete study characteristics influence study effect size by regressing effect size (dependent variable) on study characteristics (independent variables). The estimated coefficients of study characteristics and the associated statistical tests can then be used to assess whether study characteristics influence study effect sizes in a statistically significant manner. Similar to meta-analysis, there are typically two types of meta-regression. The first is random-effects meta-regression where both within-study variation and between-study variation are taken into account. The second is fixed-effects meta-regression where only within-study variation is taken into account (between-study variation is assumed to be zero). As pointed out by Normand (1999) and van Houwelingen et al. (2002), fixed-effects meta-regression is more powerful, but is less reliable if the between-study variation is significant. Therefore, random-effects meta-regression is more commonly used in the analysis which can provide a test of between-study variation (i.e. the Q-statistic from heterogeneity) along with the estimates and tests of effects of study characteristics from regression.

However, whether fixed-effects or random-effects meta-regression should be performed should be based on a detailed review of all aspects of the individual studies (see Section 3.4 of Chapter 3). Following this review if it is reasonable to believe 'a priori' that each study would provide an estimate of the same (or common) treatment effect, then a fixed-effects meta-regression model should be used. Otherwise, use a random- effects meta-regression model.

The structure of this chapter is similar to that of previous chapters. We introduce three datasets appearing in the literature in Section 7.1 to be used to illustrate the methods and R implementation. The first dataset contains summary information from 13 studies on the effectiveness of BCG vaccine against tuberculosis. The second dataset contains summary information from 28 studies on ischaemic heart disease (IHD) to assess the association between IHD risk reduction and reduction in serum cholesterol. Both datasets are widely used in meta-regression as examples. We recompiled a third dataset from Huizenga et al. (2009) to assess whether the ability to inhibit motor responses is impaired for adolescents with attention-deficit hyperactivity disorder (ADHD). We then introduce meta-regression methods in Section 7.2 and use the first dataset to illustrate these methods step-by-step. In Section 7.3, we illustrate meta-regression using the R library `metafor` for the other two datasets. We switch R library from `meta` and `rmeta` to `metafor` in this chapter since the libraries of `rmeta` and `meta` do not have the functionality of meta-regression. Some discussion is given in Section 7.4.

Note to the readers: you need to install R packages `gdata` to read in the Excel data file and `metafor` for meta-analysis.

7.1 Data

7.1.1 Bacillus Calmette-Guerin Vaccine Data

This is a dataset from clinical trials conducted to assess the impact of a Bacillus Calmette-Guerin (BCG) vaccine in the prevention of tuberculosis (TB). The dataset is widely used to illustrate meta-regression; for example, in the books authored by Everitt and Hothorn (2006) (see Table 12.2), Hartung et al. (2008) (see Table 18.8) and Borenstein et al. (2009) (see Table 20.1), as well as in the paper by van Houwelingen et al. (2002) and the R library metafor by Viechtbauer (2010). The source dataset was reported in the original publication in Colditz et al. (1994) which included 13 clinical trials of BCG vaccine each investigating the effectiveness of BCG in the treatment of tuberculosis.

It should be noticed that the numbers reported in these references are different even though all of them referenced this dataset as BCG with 13 studies from the same publications. The data tables reported from Everitt and Hothorn (2006), Borenstein et al. (2009) and Colditz et al. (1994) are the total number of cases in both BCG and control. However, the dataset reported in the R metafor library and van Houwelingen et al. (2002) are the numbers of 'negative cases'. We will use this data structure in this chapter which is given in Table 7.1.

TABLE 7.1: Data from Studies on Efficacy of BCG Vaccine for Preventing Tuberculosis.

author	year	tpos	tneg	cpos	cneg	ablat	alloc
Aronson	1948	4	119	11	128	44	random
Ferguson & Simes	1949	6	300	29	274	55	random
Rosenthal et al	1960	3	228	11	209	42	random
Hart & Sutherland	1977	62	13536	248	12619	52	random
Frimodt-Moller et al	1973	33	5036	47	5761	13	alternate
Stein & Aronson	1953	180	1361	372	1079	44	alternate
Vandiviere et al	1973	8	2537	10	619	19	random
TPT Madras	1980	505	87886	499	87892	13	random
Coetzee & Berjak	1968	29	7470	45	7232	27	random
Rosenthal et al	1961	17	1699	65	1600	42	systematic
Comstock et al	1974	186	50448	141	27197	18	systematic
Comstock & Webster	1969	5	2493	3	2338	33	systematic
Comstock et al	1976	27	16886	29	17825	33	systematic

In this table, author denotes the authorship from the 13 studies, year is publication year of these 13 studies, tpos is the number of TB positive cases in the BCG vaccinated group, tneg is the number of TB negative cases in the BCG vaccinated group, cpos is the number of TB positive cases in the control group, cneg is the number of TB negative cases in the control group, ablat denotes the absolute latitude of the study location (in degrees) and alloc denotes the method of treatment allocation with three levels of random, alternate, or systematic assignment.

The purpose of the original meta-analysis was to quantify the efficacy of the BCG vaccine against tuberculosis which was facilitated by a random-effects meta-analysis, which concluded that the BCG vaccine significantly reduced the risk of TB- in the presence of significant heterogeneity. The heterogeneity was explained partially by geographical latitude. In this chapter, we use this dataset to illustrate the application of R `metafor` library.

7.1.2 Ischaemic Heart Disease

This is a dataset from 28 randomized clinical trials of ischaemic heart disease (IHD) conducted to assess the association between IHD risk reduction and the reduction in serum cholesterol - originally analyzed in Law et al. (1994). This dataset was used by Thompson and Sharp (1999) to illustrate the increased benefit of IHD risk reduction in association with greater reduction in serum cholesterol and to explain heterogeneity in meta-analysis. The data are shown in Table 7.2 where `trial` denotes the study number from 1 to 28, with original trial reference and more detailed information listed in Law et al. (1994), `cpos` is the number of IHD events in the control group, `cneg` is the number of non-IHD event in the control group, `tpos` is the number of IHD events in the treated group, `tneg` is the number of non-IHD events in the treated group and `chol` denotes the cholesterol reduction in unit mmol/l. In this chapter, we will illustrate the application of R to analyze this dataset.

7.1.3 Attention-Deficit/Hyperactivity Disorder for Children and Adolescents

Attention-Deficit/Hyperactivity Disorder(ADHD) is one of the most common neurobehavioral disorders in children and adolescents. Typical symptoms of ADHD include difficulty staying focused and paying attention, very high levels of activity, and difficulty controlling behavior, etc. Among these symptoms, a key one is the inability to inhibit motor responses when asked to do so. There are many studies using the well-established stop-signal paradigm to measure this response in children with ADHD which typically showed a delayed stop-signal reaction time (SSRT) in comparison with healthy age-matched controls. To further study prolonged SSRT, Huizenga et al. (2009)

TABLE 7.2: Data on IHD Events from 28 Studies with Serum Cholesterol Reduction.

trial	cpos	cneg	tpos	tneg	chol
1	210	5086	173	5158	0.55
2	85	168	54	190	0.68
3	75	292	54	296	0.85
4	936	1853	676	1546	0.55
5	69	215	42	103	0.59
6	101	175	73	206	0.84
7	193	1707	157	1749	0.65
8	11	61	6	65	0.85
9	42	1087	36	1113	0.49
10	2	28	2	86	0.68
11	84	1946	54	1995	0.69
12	5	89	1	93	1.35
13	121	4395	131	4410	0.70
14	65	357	52	372	0.87
15	52	142	45	154	0.95
16	81	148	61	168	1.13
17	24	213	37	184	0.31
18	11	41	8	20	0.61
19	50	84	41	83	0.57
20	125	292	82	339	1.43
21	20	1643	62	6520	1.08
22	0	52	2	92	1.48
23	0	29	1	22	0.56
24	5	25	3	57	1.06
25	144	871	132	886	0.26
26	24	293	35	276	0.76
27	4	74	3	76	0.54
28	19	60	7	69	0.68

performed a meta-analysis of 41 studies comparing SSRT in children or adolescents diagnosed with ADHD to normal control subjects. Since between-study variation in effect sizes was large, a random-effects meta-regression analysis was conducted to investigate whether this variability could be explained by regression covariates from the between-study reaction time in "Go task" complexity. These covariates included a global index of Go task complexity measured as the mean reaction time in control subjects (RTc) and another more specific index measured as the spatial compatibility of the stimulus-response mapping.

It was found that the between-study variations were explained partially by the regression covariate RTc. There was a statistically significant relationship between the SSRT difference and RTc, where the increased SSRT difference was positively associated with increasing RTc as well as in studies that employed a noncompatible mapping compared with studies that incorporated a spatially compatible stimulus-response mapping.

In this chapter, we use R package `metafor` to analyze this data set. The data in original Table 1 and Table 2 from Huizenga et al. (2009) are re-entered into the Excel data sheet named `Data.adhd` with explanation in sheet named `readme.adhd`.

7.2 Meta-Regression

7.2.1 The Methods

As described in Section 3.2, the fundamental assumption for the fixed-effects model is that all studies share a common (true) overall effect size δ. With this assumption, the true effect size is the same (and therefore the name of fixed-effect) in all the studies with each observed effect size δ_i varying around δ with a normal sampling error; i.e. ϵ_i distributed as $N(0, \hat{\sigma}_i^2)$ where $\hat{\sigma}_i^2$ are assumed to be known.

This fundamental assumption may be impractical for some studies with substantially different effect sizes. The random-effects model relaxes this fundamental assumption by assuming (1) that the effect size $\hat{\delta}_{iR}$ from each study i

is an estimate of its own underlying true effect size δ_{iR} with sampling variance $\hat{\sigma}_i^2$, and (2) that the δ_{iR} from all studies follow an overall global distribution denoted by $N(\delta, \tau^2)$ with τ^2 as the between-study variance. If $\tau^2 = 0$, then $\delta_{1R} = \cdots = \delta_{KR} \equiv \delta$ which leads to homogeneity from all effects. In this sense, the random-effects model incorporates heterogeneity from the studies.

We have seen from Chapter 6 that even with the random-effects model, there can exist significant extra-heterogeneity. The meta-regression is then used to model this extra-heterogeneity with some study-level variables (or moderators) to account for the extra heterogeneity in the true effects. This meta-regression can be expressed as a mixed-effects model as follows:

$$\delta_{iR} = \beta_0 + \beta_1 x_{i1} + \cdots + \beta_p x_{ip} + \nu_i \tag{7.1}$$

where x_{ij} is the jth moderator variable for the ith study with associated regression parameter β_j where β_0 is the global effect size δ defined in Section 3.2 when all $\beta_1 = \cdots = \beta_p \equiv 0$. Note that ν_i is defined as $\nu_i \sim N(0, \tau^2)$ where τ^2 denotes the amount of residual heterogeneity that is not accounted for by the moderators in the meta-regression model. For this, the meta-regression is aimed to identify what moderators are significantly related to the study effects which can be used to account for the extra heterogeneity. Methodologically, the meta-regression is essentially a simple case of the general linear mixed-effects model with known heteroscedastic sampling variances provided from the study summary tables. Therefore the parameter estimation and statistical inference can be easily provided from the mixed-effects model.

We have illustrated the details for fixed-effects and random-effects models in Chapters 3, 4 and 5 using R packages `meta` and `rmeta`. These models are also implemented in R package `metafor`. Details about this package can be found in Viechtbauer (2010).

We are switching R library from `meta` and `rmeta` to `metafor` since this library includes the method of meta-regression. Readers can still use `meta` and `rmeta` for the meta-analysis following the procedures in Chapter 4 for categorical data and Chapter 5 for continuous data.

7.2.2 Example: BCG Data Analysis

7.2.2.1 Random-Effects Meta-Analysis

To use the R library, `metafor`, the original summary data from Table 7.1 have to be used to calculate the effect sizes and their associated variances. To reproduce the results from Borenstein et al. (2009) and Viechtbauer (2010), we use the same log risk ratio to estimate effect size. This effect size is a measure of the log risk ratio between the treated (i.e. vaccinated) group and control group. Hence, a negative ES indicates that BCG is favored over the control in preventing TB infection. To further promote the `metafor` library, most of the R programs in this section are modified from Viechtbauer (2010). For practice, readers can simply change `measure` from `RR` for the log risk ratio to `OR` for log odds ratio, `RD` for the risk difference, `AS` for the arcsin transformed risk difference and `PETO` for the log odds ratio estimated with Peto's method as discussed in Chapter 4 and re-run the analysis to verify.

To calculate the effect sizes using log risk ratio, we call `escalc` as follows:

```
> # Calculate the ES using "escalc"
> dat  = escalc(measure="RR",ai=tpos,bi=tneg,ci=cpos,
           di = cneg, data = dat.bcg, append = TRUE)
> # print the numerical data (Delete columns 2,3,9 to save space)
> print(dat[,-c(2,3,9)], row.names = FALSE)
```

```
 trial tpos  tneg cpos  cneg ablat      yi      vi
     1    4   119   11   128    44 -0.8893 0.32558
     2    6   300   29   274    55 -1.5854 0.19458
     3    3   228   11   209    42 -1.3481 0.41537
     4   62 13536  248 12619    52 -1.4416 0.02001
     5   33  5036   47  5761    13 -0.2175 0.05121
     6  180  1361  372  1079    44 -0.7861 0.00691
     7    8  2537   10   619    19 -1.6209 0.22302
     8  505 87886  499 87892    13  0.0120 0.00396
     9   29  7470   45  7232    27 -0.4694 0.05643
    10   17  1699   65  1600    42 -1.3713 0.07302
    11  186 50448  141 27197    18 -0.3394 0.01241
```

```
12     5  2493     3  2338      33  0.4459 0.53251
13    27 16886    29 17825      33 -0.0173 0.07140
```

It can be seen that two additonal columns are appended (resulting from the option of `append=TRUE`) to the original dataframe. They are `yi` for the effect size of log risk ratio with the corresponding (estimated) sampling variance denoted by `vi`. From this calculation, we can see that 11 out of 13 studies have a negative effect size which indicates that BCG vaccination is favored over control in preventing TB infection; i.e. the TB infection risk is lower in the BCG treatment group than in the control group in 11 of 13 studies.

To perform the meta-analysis, the function `rma` in `metafor` is called with the option `method` to specify the choice of a fixed- or a random-effects model. For the fixed-effects model, we can easily specify `method="FE"`. But for the random-effects model, there are several methods to be selected depending on which methods are to be used to estimate the between-study variance τ^2. We have extensively discussed and used the DerSimonian-Laird estimator in the previous chapter which is specified as `method="DL"` in function `rma`. Other methods implemented include:

1. `method="HS"` as the Hunter-Schmidt estimator discussed in Hunter and Schmidt (2004),

2. `method="HE"` as the Hedges estimator discussed in Hedges and Olkin (1985),

3. `method="SJ"` as the Sidik-Jonkman estimator discussed in Sidik and Jonkman (2005a) and Sidik and Jonkman (2005b),

4. `method="EB"` as the empirical Bayes estimator discussed in Morris (1983) and Berkey et al. (1995),

5. `method="ML"` and `method="REML"` as the maximum-likelihood estimator and the restricted maximum-likelihood estimator discussed in Viechtbauer (2005) with `REML` as the *default* method since `REML` is asymptotically unbiased and efficient.

The meta-analysis for the BCG data with `REML` is implemented in the following R code chunk:

```
> # Call `rma' to fit the BCG data
> meta.RE = rma(yi, vi, data = dat)
> # Print the summary
> meta.RE


Random-Effects Model (k = 13; tau^2 estimator: REML)

tau^2(estimate of total amount of heterogeneity): 0.3132(SE=0.1664)
tau (sqrt of the estimate of total heterogeneity): 0.5597
I^2 (% of total variability due to heterogeneity): 92.22%
H^2 (total variability / sampling variability):    12.86

Test for Heterogeneity:
Q(df = 12) = 152.2330, p-val < .0001

Model Results:

estimate       se     zval     pval    ci.lb    ci.ub
 -0.7145   0.1798  -3.9744   <.0001  -1.0669  -0.3622 ***

 ---
Signif. codes:  0 '***' 0.001 '**' 0.01 '*' 0.05 '.' 0.1 ' ' 1
```

From the summary, we can see that the overall effect size from a random-effects model estimated by `REML` is statistically significant (estimate= -0.7145 and p-value < 0.0001). The estimated total amount of heterogeneity $\hat{\tau}^2$ is 0.3132(SE $= 0.1664$), the percentage of total variability due to heterogeneity is $\hat{I}^2 = 92.22\%$ and the ratio of the total variability to the sampling variability is $\hat{H}^2 = 12.86$. Furthermore the `Test for Heterogeneity` is statistically significant since $\hat{Q} = 152.233$ with $df = 12$ and p-value $< .0001$. This meta-analysis can be simply summarized into the `forest` plot as shown in Figure 7.1.

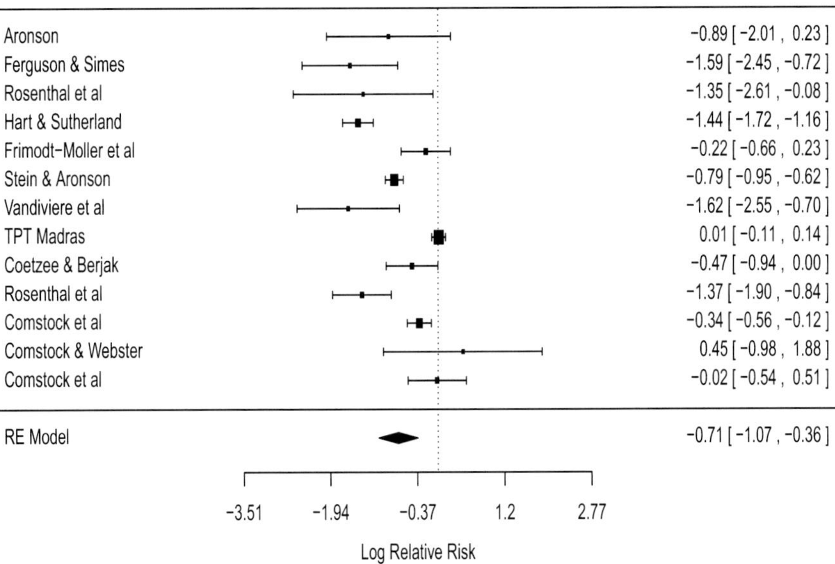

FIGURE 7.1: Forest Plot from the Random-Effects Model for BCG Data

7.2.2.2 Meta-Regression Analysis

To explain the extra-heterogeneity, we use all the moderators from the data which include `ablat`, `year` and `alloc` and call the `rma` with default `REML` method with following R code chunk:

```
> metaReg = rma(yi, vi, mods = ~ablat+year+alloc, data = dat)
> # Print the meta-regression results
> metaReg

Mixed-Effects Model (k = 13; tau^2 estimator: REML)

tau^2(estimate of residual amount of heterogeneity):0.18(SE=0.14)
tau (sqrt of the estimate of residual heterogeneity): 0.4238

Test for Residual Heterogeneity:
QE(df = 8) = 26.2030, p-val = 0.0010
Test of Moderators (coefficient(s) 2,3,4,5):
QM(df = 4) = 9.5254, p-val = 0.0492

Model Results:
                estimate      se    zval   pval   ci.lb  ci.ub
intrcpt         -14.4984 38.3943 -0.3776 0.7057 -89.7498 60.7531
ablat            -0.0236  0.0132 -1.7816 0.0748  -0.0495  0.0024 .
year              0.0075  0.0194  0.3849 0.7003  -0.0306  0.0456
allocrandom      -0.3421  0.4180 -0.8183 0.4132  -1.1613  0.4772
allocsystematic   0.0101  0.4467  0.0226 0.9820  -0.8654  0.8856
```

Although the `Test for Residual Heterogeneity` is still statistically significant ($Q_E = 26.2030$ with $df = 8$ and p-value $= 0.0010$) from this meta-regression, the estimated between-study variance dropped to 0.1796 from the previous meta-analysis of 0.3132 which indicates that (0.3132-0.1796)/0.3132 = 42.7% of the total amount of heterogeneity is accounted for by the three moderators. However, both `year` as a continuous moderator and `alloc` as a categorical moderator are highly insignificant. So we reduce the model to include only `ablat` as follows:

```
> metaReg.ablat = rma(yi, vi, mods = ~ablat, data = dat)
> # Print the meta-regression results
> metaReg.ablat

Mixed-Effects Model (k = 13; tau^2 estimator: REML)

tau^2(estimate of residual amount of heterogeneity):0.076(SE=0.06)
tau (sqrt of the estimate of residual heterogeneity): 0.2763

Test for Residual Heterogeneity:
QE(df = 11) = 30.7331, p-val = 0.0012
Test of Moderators (coefficient(s) 2):
QM(df = 1) = 16.3571, p-val < .0001

Model Results:
        estimate     se    zval   pval   ci.lb  ci.ub
intrcpt   0.2515 0.2491  1.0095 0.3127 -0.2368  0.7397
ablat    -0.0291 0.0072 -4.0444 <.0001 -0.0432 -0.0150 ***
```

As can be seen from the output, with only `ablat`, the estimated residual heterogeneity $\hat{\tau}^2$ dropped to 0.0764 (SE = 0.0591) suggesting that there is confounding among `ablat`, `year` and `alloc`. In addition, the `ablat` is more strongly statistically significant as seen from the p-value which dropped to $p < 0.0001$ as compared to $p = 0.0748$ in previous meta-regression model.

In fact, the moderator `ablat` itself accounts for (0.3132-0.0764)/0.3132 = 75.6% of the total amount of heterogeneity, and the absolute latitude is significantly related to the effectiveness of the BCG vaccine in preventing TB which can be quantified in the estimated meta-regression equation as follows:

$$log(RR) = 0.2515 - 0.0291 \times ablat \tag{7.2}$$

This estimated equation and the entire meta-regression summary can be graphically displayed in Figure 7.2 using the following R code chunk:

```
> # Create a new latitude vector
> newlat = 0:60
> # Using the meta-regression and calculate the predicted values
```

```
> preds  = predict(metaReg.ablat, newmods = newlat, transf = exp)
> # Use the inverse-variance to create a weighting for the data
> wi     = 1/sqrt(dat$vi)
> size   = 1 + 3 * (wi - min(wi))/(max(wi) - min(wi))
> # Plot the RR
> plot(dat$ablat, exp(dat$yi), pch = 19, cex = size,
  xlab = "Absolute Latitude", ylab = "Relative Risk",
  las = 1, bty = "l", log = "y")
> # Add a thicker line for the meta-regression and the CIs
> lines(newlat, preds$pred, lwd=3)
> lines(newlat, preds$ci.lb, lty = "dashed")
> lines(newlat, preds$ci.ub, lty = "dashed")
> # Add a dotted horizontal line for equal-effectiveness
> abline(h = 1, lwd=3,lty = "dotted")
```

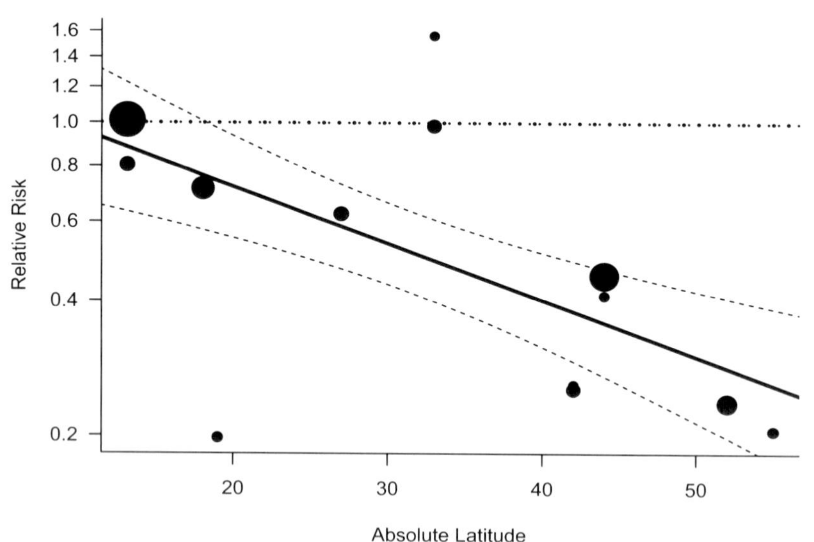

FIGURE 7.2: Meta-Regression from the Random-Effects Model for BCG

It can be seen from this equation and the associated Figure 7.2 that the higher the absolute latitude, the more effective is the BCG vaccine. When the `ablat` is less than 20 degrees and close to zero (i.e. study performed closer to equator), the effect size would be close to zero (as evidenced from the insignificant intercept parameter and Figure 7.2) which means that the vaccination has no real effect on TB. As `ablat` increases, say to a latitude of 60 degrees, the log RR as calculated from equation 7.2 is -1.49 which corresponds to a risk ratio of 0.224. In this latitude, the BCG vaccine would decrease the TB risk by 77.6% and effectively prevent the development of TB.

It should be emphasized that the `Test for Residual Heterogeneity` is still statistically significant as seen from $Q_E = 30.7331$ with $df = 11$ and p-value $= 0.0012$ which would suggest that there are more unknown moderators that impact effectiveness of the vaccine. More analyses can be performed of this dataset as seen in Viechtbauer (2010). Interested readers can reanalyze this data using other `methods` in `rma`.

7.2.3 Meta-Regression vs Weighted Regression

It is commonly regarded that the meta-regression is a version of weighted regression with the weighting factor as $w_i = \frac{1}{\hat{\sigma}_i^2 + \hat{\tau}^2}$. In this weighting factor, $\hat{\sigma}_i^2$ is the observed variance associated with the effect-size $\hat{\delta}_i$ which can be calculated using `escalc` depending on data type and different `measure` specifications whereas $\hat{\tau}^2$ is the estimated residual variance which can be obtained from `rma`.

However, if we simply call `lm` incorporating this weighting factor, the standard errors and the associated inferences (i.e. p-values) can be wrong even though the parameter estimates are correct. For example, using the meta-regression *metaReg.ablat* in the previous section, we can use the following R code chunk for illustration:

```
> # Create the weighting factor
> wi = 1/(dat$vi+metaReg.ablat$tau2)
> # Call `lm' for weighted regression
> weightedReg = lm(yi~ablat, data=dat, weights=wi)
> # Print the summary
> summary(weightedReg)
```

```
Call:
lm(formula = yi ~ ablat, data = dat, weights = wi)

Residuals:
   Min     1Q Median     3Q    Max
-2.412 -0.538 -0.225  0.490  1.799

Coefficients:
            Estimate Std. Error t value Pr(>|t|)
(Intercept)   0.2515     0.2839    0.89   0.3948
ablat        -0.0291     0.0082   -3.55   0.0046 **

Residual standard error: 1.14 on 11 degrees of freedom
Multiple R-squared: 0.534,      Adjusted R-squared: 0.491
F-statistic: 12.6 on 1 and 11 DF,  p-value: 0.00457
```

Comparing this output with the output from *metaReg.ablat* from the above subsection, we can see that the parameter estimates are the same as $\hat{\beta}_0$ for `intercept` = 0.2515 and $\hat{\beta}_1$ for `ablat` = -0.0291. However the estimated standard errors and p-values are all different.

So what is wrong? The key to making correct inferences is from the model specification. In meta-regression, the model is assumed to be

$$y_i = \beta_0 + \beta_1 x_{i1} + \cdots + \beta_p x_{pi} + e_i \tag{7.3}$$

where $e_i \sim N(0, w_i)$ with known w_i. However in the weighted regression as illustrated in *weightedReg*, the model assumed seems to be the same as

$$y_i = \beta_0 + \beta_1 x_{i1} + \cdots + \beta_p x_{pi} + e_i \tag{7.4}$$

However the error distribution by default is $e_i \sim N(0, \sigma^2 \times w_i)$. `lm` will then estimate σ^2 which can be seen from the ANOVA table to be $\hat{\sigma} = 1.14$. With meta-regression, this σ^2 should set to 1.

With this notation, the correct standard error would be estimated as $se(\hat{\beta}) = \sqrt{H_w}$ for the meta-regression instead of the $se(\hat{\beta}) = \hat{\sigma} \times \sqrt{H_w}$ from the weighted linear model. From this correct standard error, appropriate inference can then be made. This procedure can be more explicitly illustrated by the following R code chunk:

```
> # Take the response vector
> y = dat$yi
> # Make the design matrix
> X = cbind(1,dat$ablat)
> # Make the weight matrix
> W = diag(wi)
> # Calculate the parameter estimate
> betahat = solve(t(X)%*%W%*%X)%*%t(X)%*%W%*%y
> # Calculate the estimated variance
> var.betahat =  diag(solve(t(X)%*%W%*%X))
> # Calculate the standard error
> se.betahat = sqrt(var.betahat)
> # Calculate z-value assuming asymptotic normal
> z = betahat/se.betahat
> # Calculate the p-value
> pval = 2*(1-pnorm(abs(z)))
> # Calculate the 95% CI
> ci.lb = betahat-1.96*se.betahat
> ci.ub = betahat+1.96*se.betahat
> # Make the output similar to metaReg.ablat
> Mod.Results = cbind(betahat, se.betahat,z,pval,ci.lb,ci.ub)
> colnames(Mod.Results) = c("estimate", "se","zval","pval",
                            "ci.lb","ci.ub")
> rownames(Mod.Results) = c("intrcpt", "ablat")
> # Print the result
> round(Mod.Results,4)
```

```
        estimate     se  zval   pval   ci.lb  ci.ub
intrcpt   0.2515 0.2491  1.01 0.3127 -0.2368  0.740
ablat    -0.0291 0.0072 -4.04 0.0001 -0.0432 -0.015
```

This reproduces the results from `metaReg.ablat`.

7.3 Data Analysis Using R

7.3.1 IHD Data Analysis

The data in Table 7.2 were recompiled and typed into the Excel data book with data sheet named as `Data.IHD` which can be loaded into R using following R code chunk:

```
> # Load the library
> require(gdata)
> # Get the data path
> datfile = "Your Data Path/dat4Meta.xls"
> # Call "read.xls" to read the Excel data sheet
> dat.IHD  = read.xls(datfile, sheet="Data.IHD",
                         perl="c:/perl64/bin/perl.exe")
```

It should be noted that there are two 0's in `cpos` for trials 22 and 23. In performing the meta-analysis and meta-regression, 0.5 is added to these two 0's.

7.3.1.1 Random-Effects Meta-Analysis

To reproduce the results from Thompson and Sharp (1999), we use the same log odds-ratios in this section as the measure for the effect sizes. To calculate the effect sizes using log odds-ratio, we can call `escalc` as follows:

```
> # Calculate the ES using "escalc"
> dat  = escalc(measure="OR",ai=tpos,bi=tneg,ci=cpos,
         di = cneg, data = dat.IHD, append = TRUE)
> # print the numerical data
> print(dat, row.names = FALSE)

 trial cpos cneg tpos tneg chol     yi      vi
     1  210 5086  173 5158 0.55 -0.208 0.01093
     2   85  168   54  190 0.68 -0.577 0.04150
     3   75  292   54  296 0.85 -0.342 0.03865
     4  936 1853  676 1546 0.55 -0.144 0.00373
```

```
5   69  215  42  103 0.59  0.239 0.05266
6  101  175  73  206 0.84 -0.488 0.03417
7  193 1707 157 1749 0.65 -0.231 0.01271
8   11   61   6   65 0.85 -0.670 0.28935
9   42 1087  36 1113 0.49 -0.178 0.05341
10   2   28   2   86 0.68 -1.122 1.04734
11  84 1946  54 1995 0.69 -0.467 0.03144
12   5   89   1   93 1.35 -1.653 1.22199
13 121 4395 131 4410 0.70  0.076 0.01635
14  65  357  52  372 0.87 -0.264 0.04010
15  52  142  45  154 0.95 -0.226 0.05499
16  81  148  61  168 1.13 -0.410 0.04145
17  24  213  37  184 0.31  0.579 0.07882
18  11   41   8   20 0.61  0.399 0.29030
19  50   84  41   83 0.57 -0.186 0.06834
20 125  292  82  339 1.43 -0.571 0.02657
21  20 1643  62 6520 1.08 -0.247 0.06689
22   0   52   2   92 1.48  1.043 2.42986
23   0   29   1   22 0.56  1.369 2.74501
24   5   25   3   57 1.06 -1.335 0.59088
25 144  871 132  886 0.26 -0.104 0.01680
26  24  293  35  276 0.76  0.437 0.07727
27   4   74   3   76 0.54 -0.314 0.61000
28  19   60   7   69 0.68 -1.138 0.22665
```

Two additional columns are appended (resulting from the option `append=TRUE`) to the original dataframe where column `yi` is the effect size for log odds-ratio with the corresponding (estimated) sampling variance denoted by column `vi`. Pay special attention to trial numbers 22 and 23 where 0.5 was added as control events in order to calculate the log odds-ratio and the variances, resulting in log odds-ratios of 1.043 and 1.369 with large variances of 2.4299 and 2.7450, respectively.

The meta-analysis with default `REML` is implemented in the following R code chunk:

```
> # Call `rma' to fit the BCG data
> meta.RE = rma(yi, vi, data = dat)
> # Print the summary
> meta.RE


Random-Effects Model (k = 28; tau^2 estimator: REML)


tau^2(estimate of total amount of heterogeneity):0.03(SE=0.02)
tau (sqrt of the estimate of total heterogeneity): 0.1790
I^2 (% of total variability due to heterogeneity): 47.77%
H^2 (total variability / sampling variability):    1.91


Test for Heterogeneity:
Q(df = 27) = 49.9196, p-val = 0.0046


Model Results:


estimate      se     zval    pval    ci.lb    ci.ub
 -0.2193 0.0571 -3.8401 0.0001 -0.3312 -0.1074 ***
---
Signif. codes:  0 '***' 0.001 '**' 0.01 '*' 0.05 '.' 0.1 ' ' 1
```

From the summary, we can see that the overall effect-size from a random-effects model estimated by REML is statistically significant (estimate= -0.2193 and p-value $= 0.0001$). The estimated total amount of heterogeneity $\hat{\tau}^2$ is $0.0321(\text{SE} = 0.0207)$, the percentage of total variability due to heterogeneity is $\hat{I}^2 = 47.77\%$ and the ratio of the total variability to the sampling variability is $\hat{H}^2 = 1.91$. Furthermore the Test for Heterogeneity is statistically significant since $\hat{Q} = 49.9196$ with $df = 27$ and p-value $=0.0046$.

7.3.1.2 Meta-Regression Analysis

To explain the extra-heterogeneity, we use the cholesterol reduction (chol) as a moderator and call the rma for a meta-regression analysis using the following R code chunk:

```
> metaReg.RE.REML = rma(yi, vi, mods = ~chol, data = dat)
> # Print the meta-regression results
> metaReg.RE.REML

Mixed-Effects Model (k = 28; tau^2 estimator: REML)

tau^2(estimate of residual amount of heterogeneity):0.0107(SE=0.0122)
tau (sqrt of the estimate of residual heterogeneity): 0.1035

Test for Residual Heterogeneity:
QE(df = 26) = 38.2448, p-val = 0.0575
Test of Moderators (coefficient(s) 2):
QM(df = 1) = 8.9621, p-val = 0.0028

Model Results:
       estimate     se    zval   pval   ci.lb  ci.ub
intrcpt  0.1389 0.1258  1.1037 0.2697 -0.1078  0.3855
chol    -0.5013 0.1675 -2.9937 0.0028 -0.8295 -0.1731 **
```

It can be seen from this meta-regression that the `Test for Residual Heterogeneity` is no longer statistically significant at the 5%-level ($Q_E = 38.2448$ with $df = 26$ and p-value $= 0.0575$). The estimated between-study variance dropped to 0.0107 from the previous meta-analysis of 0.0321 which indicates that (0.0321-0.0107)/0.0321 = 66.7% of the total amount of heterogeneity is accounted for by the cholesterol reduction with estimated meta-regression equation as:

$$log(OR) = 0.1389 - 0.5013 \times chol \tag{7.5}$$

This estimated equation and the entire meta-regression summary is graphically displayed in Figure 7.3 using the following R code chunk:

```
> # Create a new cholesterol reduction vector
> newx   = seq(0,1.5, length=100)
> # Using the meta-regression and calculate the predicted values
> preds  =  predict(metaReg.RE.REML, newmods = newx, transf=exp)
> # Use the inverse-variance to create a weighting for the data
```

```
> wi      =  1/sqrt(dat$vi+metaReg.RE.REML$tau2)
> size    =  1 + 2*(wi - min(wi))/(max(wi) - min(wi))
> # Plot the OR
> plot(dat$chol, exp(dat$yi),pch = 1,cex = size, xlim=c(0, 1.6),
  ylim=c(0,2), las = 1, bty = "l", ylab = "Odds Ratio",
  xlab = "Absolute Reduction in Cholesterol (mmol/l)")
> # Add a thicker line for the meta-regression and CIs
> lines(newx, preds$pred, lwd=3)
> lines(newx, preds$ci.lb, lty = "dashed")
> lines(newx, preds$ci.ub, lty = "dashed")
> # Add a dotted horizontal line for equal-effectiveness
> abline(h = 1, lwd=3,lty = "dotted")
```

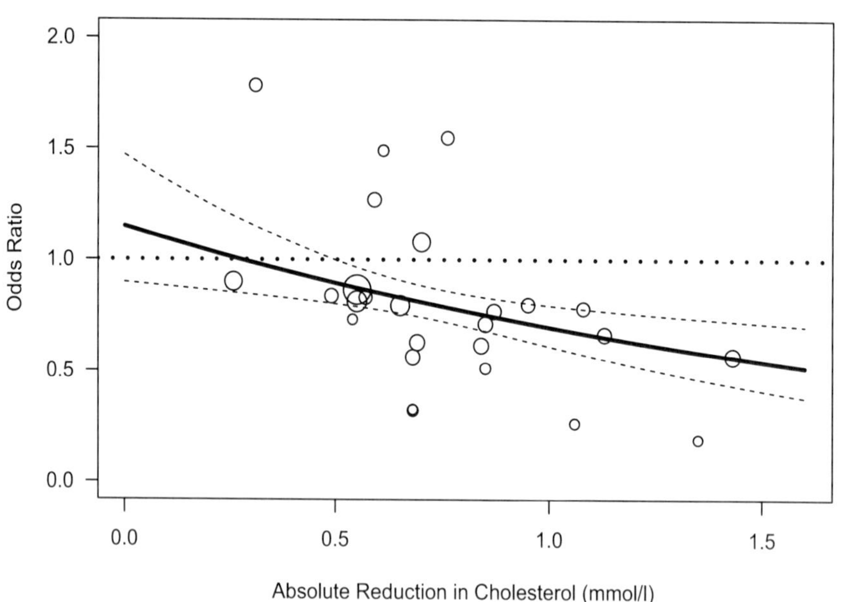

FIGURE 7.3: Meta-Regression from the Random-Effects Model for IHD Data

7.3.1.3 Comparison of Different Fitting Methods

As pointed in Section 7.2.2.1, there are several methods in `rma` for fitting a fixed- or a random-effects model. The `method="FE"` is for fixed-effects models. For random-effects models, there are choices to estimate the variance τ^2; i.e. the DerSimonian-Laird estimator specified as `method="DL"`, the Hunter-Schmidt estimator specified as `method="HS"`, the Hedges estimator specified as `method="HE"`, the Sidik-Jonkman estimator specified as `method="SJ"`, the empirical Bayes estimator specified as `method="EB"`, the maximum-likelihood estimator specified as `method="ML"` and the restricted maximum-likelihood estimator specified as `method="REML"`. Different methods to estimate τ^2 will impact outcomes from the meta-regression. We are illustrating this impact using the ICH data which can be easily implemented as in the following R code chunk:

```
> # The fixed-effects meta-regression
> metaReg.FE = rma(yi, vi, mods= ~chol,data=dat,method="FE")
> metaReg.FE

Fixed-Effects with Moderators Model (k = 28)

Test for Residual Heterogeneity:
QE(df = 26) = 38.2448, p-val = 0.0575
Test of Moderators (coefficient(s) 2):
QM(df = 1) = 11.6748, p-val = 0.0006

Model Results:
        estimate     se     zval   pval   ci.lb  ci.ub
intrcpt   0.1153 0.0972  1.1861 0.2356 -0.0752  0.3059
chol     -0.4723 0.1382 -3.4168 0.0006 -0.7432 -0.2014 ***
 ---
Signif. codes:  0 '***' 0.001 '**' 0.01 '*' 0.05 '.' 0.1 ' ' 1

> # The random-effects meta-regression with "DL"
> metaReg.RE.DL = rma(yi,vi,mods=~chol,data=dat,method="DL")
> metaReg.RE.DL
```

```
Mixed-Effects Model (k = 28; tau^2 estimator: DL)

tau^2 (estimate of residual amount of heterogeneity): 0.0170
tau (sqrt of the estimate of residual heterogeneity): 0.1305

Test for Residual Heterogeneity:
QE(df = 26) = 38.2448, p-val = 0.0575
Test of Moderators (coefficient(s) 2):
QM(df = 1) = 8.0471, p-val = 0.0046

Model Results:
        estimate     se    zval   pval   ci.lb   ci.ub
intrcpt   0.1491 0.1378  1.0826 0.2790 -0.1209  0.4192
chol     -0.5137 0.1811 -2.8367 0.0046 -0.8686 -0.1588 **

---
Signif. codes:  0 '***' 0.001 '**' 0.01 '*' 0.05 '.' 0.1 ' ' 1

> # The random-effects meta-regression with "HS"
> metaReg.RE.HS = rma(yi,vi,mods=~chol,data=dat,method="HS")
> metaReg.RE.HS

Mixed-Effects Model (k = 28; tau^2 estimator: HS)

tau^2 (estimate of residual amount of heterogeneity): 0.0116
tau (sqrt of the estimate of residual heterogeneity): 0.1076

Test for Residual Heterogeneity:
QE(df = 26) = 38.2448, p-val = 0.0575
Test of Moderators (coefficient(s) 2):
QM(df = 1) = 8.8185, p-val = 0.0030

Model Results:
        estimate     se    zval   pval   ci.lb   ci.ub
intrcpt   0.1404 0.1276  1.1005 0.2711 -0.1097  0.3905
chol     -0.5032 0.1694 -2.9696 0.0030 -0.8353 -0.1711**
```

```
---
Signif. codes:  0 '***' 0.001 '**' 0.01 '*' 0.05 '.' 0.1 ' ' 1

> # The random-effects meta-regression with "HE"
> metaReg.RE.HE = rma(yi,vi,mods=~chol,data=dat,method="HE")
> metaReg.RE.HE

Mixed-Effects Model (k = 28; tau^2 estimator: HE)

tau^2 (estimate of residual amount of heterogeneity): 0.0618
tau (sqrt of the estimate of residual heterogeneity): 0.2486

Test for Residual Heterogeneity:
QE(df = 26) = 38.2448, p-val = 0.0575
Test of Moderators (coefficient(s) 2):
QM(df = 1) = 5.0345, p-val = 0.0248

Model Results:
        estimate     se     zval    pval    ci.lb   ci.ub
intrcpt   0.1895 0.1962   0.9661 0.3340 -0.1950  0.5741
chol     -0.5647 0.2517  -2.2438 0.0248 -1.0579 -0.0714 *
---
Signif. codes:  0 '***' 0.001 '**' 0.01 '*' 0.05 '.' 0.1 ' ' 1

> # The random-effects meta-regression with "SJ"
> metaReg.RE.SJ = rma(yi,vi,mods=~chol,data=dat,method="SJ")
> metaReg.RE.SJ

Mixed-Effects Model (k = 28; tau^2 estimator: SJ)

tau^2 (estimate of residual amount of heterogeneity): 0.1389
tau (sqrt of the estimate of residual heterogeneity): 0.3727

Test for Residual Heterogeneity:
QE(df = 26) = 38.2448, p-val = 0.0575
Test of Moderators (coefficient(s) 2):
QM(df = 1) = 3.3004, p-val = 0.0693
```

```
Model Results:
        estimate      se     zval    pval    ci.lb   ci.ub
intrcpt   0.2169 0.2619   0.8279 0.4077 -0.2966 0.7303
chol     -0.6053 0.3332 -1.8167 0.0693 -1.2584 0.0477 .
 ---
Signif. codes:  0 '***' 0.001 '**' 0.01 '*' 0.05 '.' 0.1 ' ' 1

> # The random-effects meta-regression with "ML"
> metaReg.RE.ML = rma(yi,vi,mods=~chol,data=dat,method="ML")
> metaReg.RE.ML

Mixed-Effects Model (k = 28; tau^2 estimator: ML)

tau^2(estimate of residual amount of heterogeneity):0.00(SE=0.0045)
tau (sqrt of the estimate of residual heterogeneity): 0.0022

Test for Residual Heterogeneity:
QE(df = 26) = 38.2448, p-val = 0.0575
Test of Moderators (coefficient(s) 2):
QM(df = 1) = 11.6726, p-val = 0.0006

Model Results:
        estimate      se     zval    pval    ci.lb   ci.ub
intrcpt   0.1153 0.0972   1.1860 0.2356 -0.0753  0.3059
chol     -0.4723 0.1382 -3.4165 0.0006 -0.7432 -0.2013  ***
---
Signif. codes:  0 '***' 0.001 '**' 0.01 '*' 0.05 '.' 0.1 ' ' 1

> # The random-effects meta-regression with "EB"
> metaReg.RE.EB = rma(yi,vi,mods=~chol,data=dat,method="EB")
> metaReg.RE.EB

Mixed-Effects Model (k = 28; tau^2 estimator: EB)

tau^2 (estimate of residual amount of heterogeneity): 0.0299
tau (sqrt of the estimate of residual heterogeneity): 0.1730
```

```
Test for Residual Heterogeneity:
QE(df = 26) = 38.2448, p-val = 0.0575
Test of Moderators (coefficient(s) 2):
QM(df = 1) = 6.7671, p-val = 0.0093

Model Results:
        estimate     se    zval    pval   ci.lb   ci.ub
intrcpt   0.1651 0.1579  1.0454 0.2958 -0.1444  0.4746
chol     -0.5331 0.2049 -2.6014 0.0093 -0.9348 -0.1314  **
 ---
Signif. codes:  0 '***' 0.001 '**' 0.01 '*' 0.05 '.' 0.1 ' ' 1
```

We summarize the results from this series of model fittings along with the meta-analysis in Section 7.3.1.1 and the meta-regression in Section 7.3.1.2 in Table 7.3.

TABLE 7.3: Summary of Model Fittings

Method	Intercept(SE)	Slope(SE)	$\hat{\tau}^2$	$\hat{Q}$	p-value
Meta	-0.219(0.057)	NA	0.032	49.920	0.005
FE	0.115(0.097)	-0.472(0.138)	0.000	38.245	0.057
RE.DL	0.149(0.138)	-0.514(0.181)	0.017	38.245	0.057
RE.HS	0.140(0.128)	-0.503(0.169)	0.012	38.245	0.057
RE.HE	0.190(0.196)	-0.565(0.252)	0.062	38.245	0.057
RE.SJ	0.217(0.262)	-0.605(0.333)	0.139	38.245	0.057
RE.ML	0.115(0.097)	-0.472(0.138)	0.000	38.245	0.057
RE.EB	0.165(0.158)	-0.533(0.205)	0.030	38.245	0.057
RE.REML	0.139(0.126)	-0.501(0.167)	0.011	38.245	0.057

In this table, the column "Method" denotes the fitting method with the first "Meta" for meta-analysis in Section 7.3.1.1, "FE" for fixed-effect meta-regression and the next seven for random-effects regression analyses (prefixed with "RE"). The second and third columns are the estimated intercept and slope along with their standard errors from the meta-regression. Notice that for meta-analysis (i.e. the first row) there is no estimated slope parameter which is denoted by "NA". The column labeled $\hat{\tau}^2$ is the estimated between (residual)-variance where $\hat{\tau}^2 = 0$ is for fixed-effects (i.e. "FE") meta-regression. The last two columns are for the estimated heterogeneity (Q) quantity and its associated p-value from the χ^2-test and they are the same for all meta-regressions since $\hat{Q}$ is independent of the $\hat{\tau}^2$. From this table, we can see that the estimates for the parameters and between-study variance are slightly different. However, the fundamental conclusion is the same; i.e. there is a statistically significant relationship between the serum cholesterol reduction and IHD risk reduction.

Similar analyses can be performed by using different measures of study effects. For this data, we used log odds-ratio. Other possible choices are Peto's log odds-ratio, log relative risk, risk difference and the arcsin transformed risk difference. Analyses can be performed with the library `metafor`, using the function `escalc` to specify `measure=PETO` for Peto's log odds-ratio, `measure=RR` for log relative risk, `measure=RD` for risk difference and `measure=AS` for the arcsin transformed risk difference. We leave these as exercises for interested readers.

7.3.2 ADHD Data Analysis

7.3.2.1 Data and Variables

The data can be loaded into R using library `gdata` as follows:

```
> # Load the library
> require(gdata)
> # Get the data path
> datfile = "Your Data Path/dat4Meta.xls"
> # Call "read.xls" to read the Excel data sheet
> dat  = read.xls(datfile, sheet="Data.adhd",
                          perl="c:/perl64/bin/perl.exe")
> # Print the dimmension of the dataframe
> dim(dat)

[1] 41 26
```

The dependent variable was chosen as the SSRT difference between ADHD and control subjects with the associated variance (named as `ssrt12ssrtc` and `var.ssrta2ssrtc` in the dataframe). Two variables were chosen to be the independent variables for the meta-regression. One is the reaction time in the control (i.e. `crt`) which is a global index indicator of Go task complexity and is continuous. The other independent variable is the spatial compatibility (named as `cmp`) which is a more specific index of stimulus-response mapping in the Go task and is nominal variable with '-1' as 'spatially noncompatible' and '1' as 'spatially compatible'.

7.3.2.2 Meta-Analysis

We first look into the SSRT difference between ADHD and control subjects which can be implemented into `metafor` as meta-regression without independent variables. The R code chunk is as follows:

```
> # Call `rma' from metafor for default random-effect MA
> metareg.No = rma(ssrta2ssrtc,var.ssrta2ssrtc, data = dat)
> # Print the summary
> metareg.No

Random-Effects Model (k = 41; tau^2 estimator: REML)


tau^2(estimate of total amount of heterogeneity):349(SE=239.28)
tau (sqrt of the estimate of total heterogeneity): 18.6831
I^2 (% of total variability due to heterogeneity): 32.87%
H^2 (total variability / sampling variability):    1.49


Test for Heterogeneity:
Q(df = 40) = 63.4688, p-val = 0.0105


Model Results:
estimate     se    zval    pval   ci.lb   ci.ub
 67.3725 5.4115 12.4499  <.0001 56.7662 77.9789 ***
```

From the summary, we can see that the average SSRT difference between ADHD and control is 67.37 which is statistically significantly different from zero (p-value < 0.001). Furthermore, a statistically significant variation between studies was found as indicated by the heterogeneity statistic Q=63.4688 with df of 40 and p-value $= 0.0105$.

Readers can use R library `rmeta` or `meta` to reproduce these results and we leave this as practice for interested readers.

7.3.2.3 Meta-Regression Analysis

To identify the sources of heterogeneity, a meta-regression between SSRT difference and task complexity as assessed by RTc can be conducted to explain the extra-heterogeneity. The R implementation can be done using the R code chunk as follows:

```
> # Meta-regression to RTc
> metareg.crt <- rma(ssrta2ssrtc,var.ssrta2ssrtc,
                   mods =~crt, data = dat)
> # Print the summary
> metareg.crt

Mixed-Effects Model (k = 35; tau^2 estimator: REML)

tau^2(estimate of residual amount of heterogeneity):218(SE=230.06)
tau (sqrt of the estimate of residual heterogeneity): 14.7977

Test for Residual Heterogeneity:
QE(df = 33) = 44.8954, p-val = 0.0811
Test of Moderators (coefficient(s) 2):
QM(df = 1) = 3.4841, p-val = 0.0620

Model Results:
       estimate      se    zval    pval     ci.lb   ci.ub
intrcpt 16.8440 24.4404 0.6892 0.4907 -31.0583 64.7463
crt       0.0779  0.0417 1.8666 0.0620   -0.003  90.1597  .
```

A great feature for this `metafor` library is the plotting functionality which can be used to display the typical forest plot, residual funnel plot and other residual plots by simply calling the `plot` command as follows to produce Figure 7.4:

```
> # Plot all from this meta-regression
> plot(metareg.crt)
```

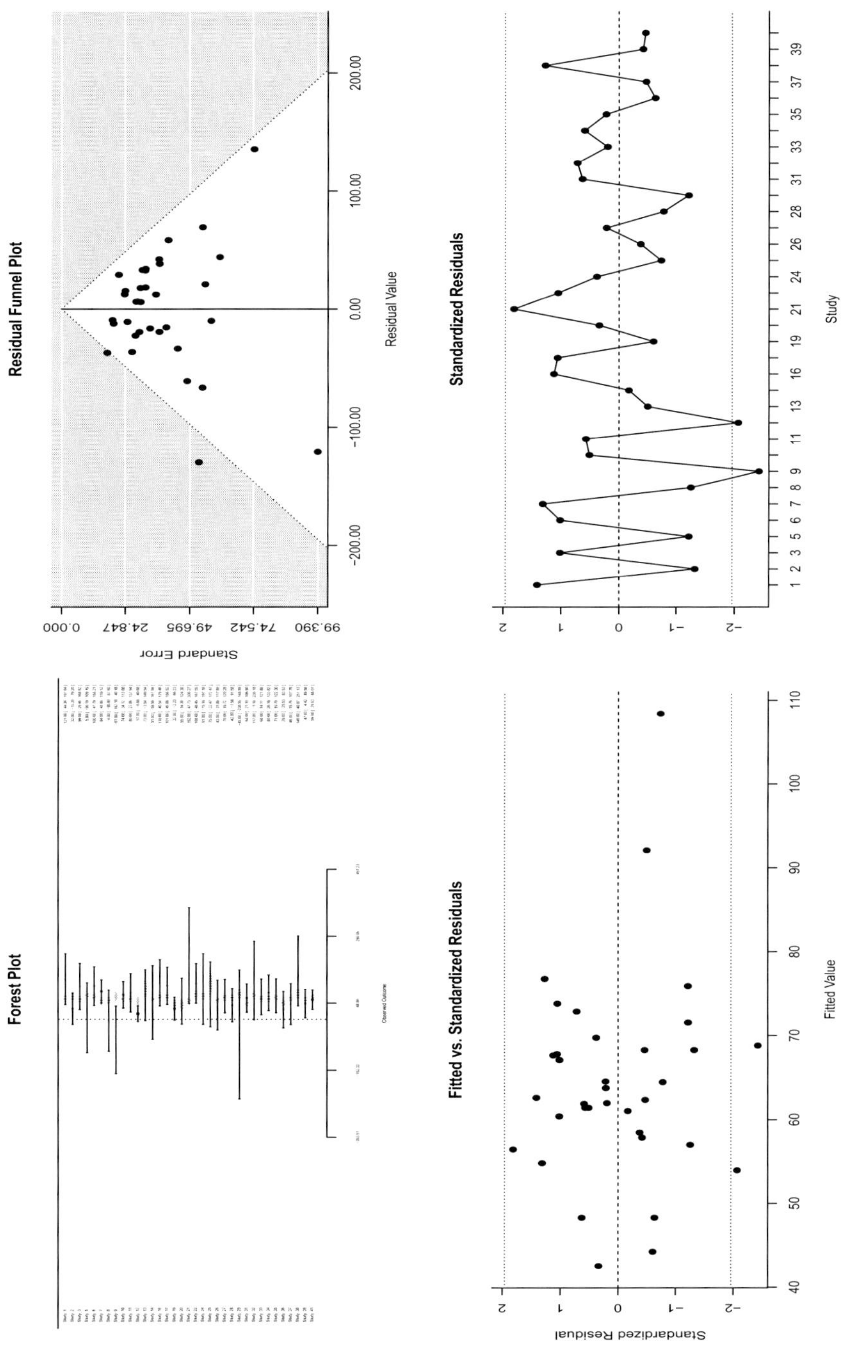

FIGURE 7.4: All Plots from the Meta-Regression

We can see from these figures again that the SSRT difference between ADHD and control are statistically significantly larger than zero. The funnel plot and the two other residual plots indicate symmetry and no systematic deviations. From the summary of the meta-regression, we can conclude that there is a positive regression ($\hat{\beta} = 0.0779$ with p-value $= 0.0620$) between the SSRT difference and the task complexity as measured by RTc. With this meta-regression, the heterogeneity statistic is now reduced to $Q = 44.8954$ which is now statistically nonsignificant (p-value $= 0.0811$). This relationship can be graphically illustrated in Figure 7.5 using the following R code chunk:

```
> plot(ssrta2ssrtc~crt, las=1, xlab="RTc",
        ylab="SSRTa-SSRTc",data = dat)
> # Add the meta-regression line to the plot
> abline(metareg.crt$b, lwd=2)
> # Fill `spatilly compatible'
> points(ssrta2ssrtc~crt,data=dat[dat$cmp==1,], pch=16)
```

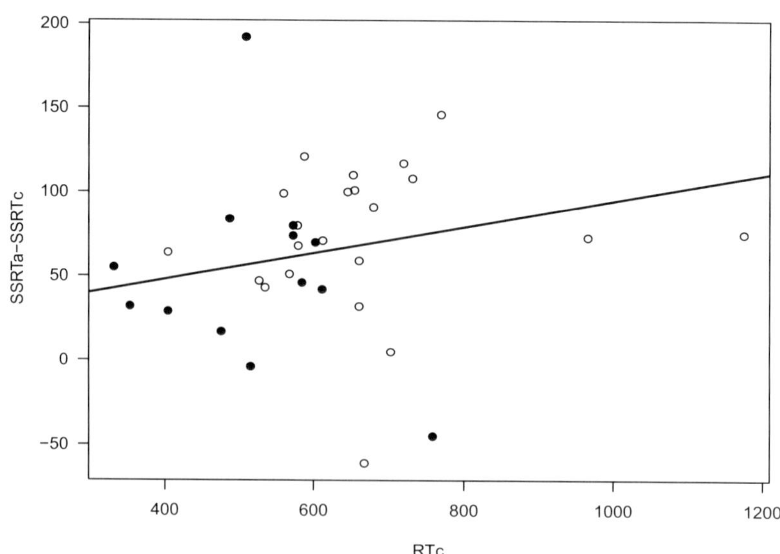

FIGURE 7.5: Reproduction of Figure 1 in the Original Paper

Figure 7.5 is a reproduction of Figure 1 in the original paper for stop-signal reaction time differences between subjects with ADHD and control subjects as a function of RTc for studies with spatially compatible (filled circles) versus a noncompatible mapping (open circles). From this figure, a positive relationship between the SSRT difference and RTc can be seen graphically which is consistent with the meta-regression summary from the above analysis. In addition, it can be seen from this figure that small SSRT differences are associated with spatially compatible responses as denoted by the filled circles and large SSRT differences with noncompatible responses as denoted by the open circles.

This observation can be statistically tested by meta-regression using the following R code chunk:

```
> # Meta-regression to spatially compatible response
> metareg.cmp = rma(ssrta2ssrtc,var.ssrta2ssrtc,
        mods =~cmp, data = dat)
> # Print the summary
> metareg.cmp

Mixed-Effects Model (k = 41; tau^2 estimator: REML)

tau^2(estimate of residual amount of heterogeneity):210(SE= 02.79)
tau (sqrt of the estimate of residual heterogeneity): 14.5060

Test for Residual Heterogeneity:
QE(df = 39) = 51.3191, p-val = 0.0895

Test of Moderators (coefficient(s) 2):
QM(df = 1) = 6.8837, p-val = 0.0087

Model Results:
       estimate     se    zval   pval    ci.lb   ci.ub
intrcpt 63.9132 5.0850 12.5691 <.0001  53.9469 73.8795 ***
cmp    -13.3413 5.0850 -2.6237 0.0087 -23.3076 -3.3750 **
```

```
---
Signif. codes:  0 '***' 0.001 '**' 0.01 '*' 0.05 '.' 0.1 ' ' 1
```

It can be seen from the summary that there was indeed a statistically significant relationship with spatial compatibility (slope estimate of $\hat{\beta} = 13.34$ and p-value $= 0.0087$). Incorporating this spatial compatibility effect into meta-regression as an independent variable reduced between-study variation; the heterogeneity statistic $Q = 51.32$ as compared to the original Q of 63.4688. With this independent variable, the test of heterogeneity is statistically significant (p-value$= 0.0087$).

To include all the meta-regression results into Figure 7.6, a better presentation can be produced with the following R code chunk as follows:

```
> # Create a new data series to cover the range of RTc
> new.crt = 300:1200
> # Calculate the predict values and the CI from the MR
> preds   = predict(metareg.crt, newmods = new.crt)
> # Create the weights for the size circles
> wi      = 1/sqrt(dat$var.ssrta2ssrtc)
> # Create the size of circles
> size    = 1+2*(wi - min(wi))/(max(wi) - min(wi))
> # Make the plot
> plot(ssrta2ssrtc~crt, las=1, xlab="RTc", cex=size,
                          ylab="SSRTa-SSRTc",data = dat)
> # Add the regression line
> abline(metareg.crt$b, lwd=2)
> # Use filled circles for `spatially compatibility
> points(ssrta2ssrtc~crt,data=dat[dat$cmp==1,], cex=size,pch=16)
> # Add CIs
> lines(new.crt, preds$ci.lb, lty = "dashed")
> lines(new.crt, preds$ci.ub, lty = "dashed")
> # Add the significant line
> abline(h = 1, lty = "dotted", lwd=3)
```

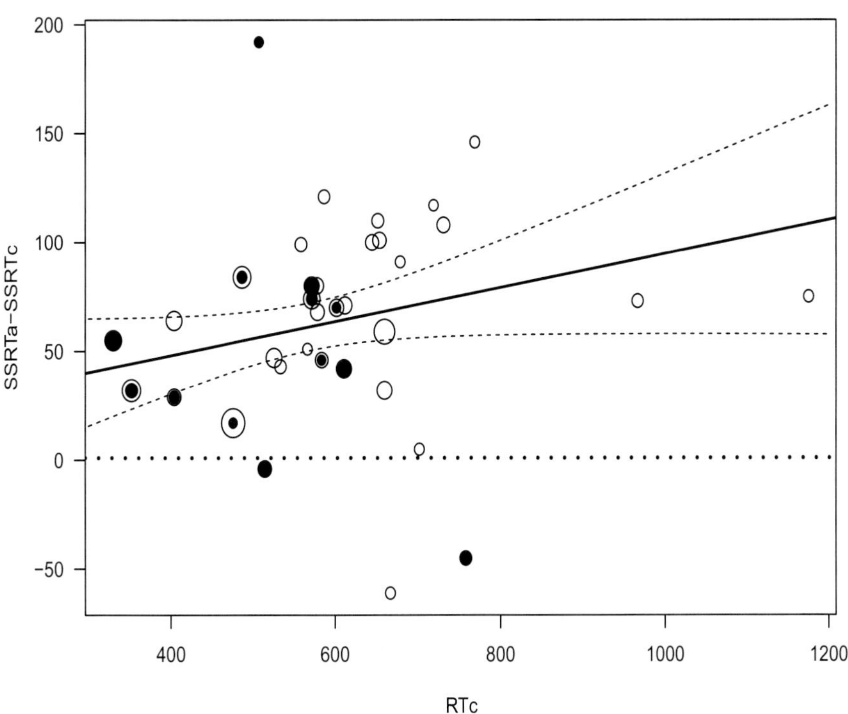

FIGURE 7.6: The Summary Plot for the Data and the Meta-Regression

7.3.2.4 Summary

Readers can see that we have reproduced the results from Huizenga et al. (2009) that SSRT for ADHD subjects was significantly higher than for normal control subjects, and task complexity was significantly related to SSRT differences and explained part of the heterogeneity. In practice, these differences could be related to other variables as seen from the data. Huizenga et al. (2009) discussed further tests for potential confounders and we leave this further analysis to interested readers as practice.

7.4 Discussion

In this chapter, we discussed meta-regression to use study-level moderators to account for extra-heterogeneity in meta-analysis. The methods for meta-regression are essentially a special case of regression with weightings obtained from within-study and between-study which can be fixed-effects and random-effects models. With meta-regression models, we can quantify the relationship between study effect-sizes and extra study moderators and test their statistical significance.

We illustrated the models used in meta-regression with three datasets from the literature using the R library `metafor`. We showed how straightforward it is to use this library for any kind of meta-regression as well as meta-analysis.

There are many references and books discussing methods and applications in meta-regression. The purpose of this chapter is to illustrate these developed methodologies and their step-by-step implementation in R. Interested readers can follow the steps and reuse the R for their own research and meta-regression analysis.

We have referred to some books and publications in this chapter. We further recommend the paper by Thompson and Higgins (2002) and the books by Roberts and Stanley (2005), Petitti (2000) and Pigott (2012) to readers.

Chapter 8

Individual-Patient Level Data Analysis versus Meta-Analysis

There are extensive discussions about the relative merits of performing individual-patient level data (IPD) analysis versus meta-analysis (MA) in those cases where IPD are accessible. Some favor IPD and others favor MA. In this chapter we use placebo controlled clinical studies of lamotrigine in the treatment of bipolar depression to illustrate the pros and cons of IPD and MA. Two clinical outcome measures, the Hamilton Rating Scale for Depression (HAMD) and the Montgomery-Asberg Depression Rating Scale (MADRS), are used. This chapter is organized as follows. In Section 8.1 we introduce this data as well as the descriptive statistics for the data. We then present data analysis from both IPD and MA on treatment comparison for changes in HAMD in Section 8.2 and changes in MADRS in Section 8.3 - both of which led to the same conclusions as summarized in Section 8.4. Based on these conclusions, we then formulate a simulation to compare the efficiency of IPD to MA in Section 8.5 followed by discussion in Section 8.6.

8.1 Introduction

In Chapter 4, we referred to a meta-analysis using five studies of Lamotrigine in the treatment of bipolar depression which was analyzed by Geddes et al. (2009). The studies were conducted by GlaxoSmithKline. We requested the individual patient-level data from the company so that we can use the data in this chapter to illustrate the IPD and meta-analysis.

Five studies were reported in Geddes et al. (2009) as Study 1

(GW602/SCAB2001), Study 2 (GW603/SCAA2010), Study 3 (SCA40910), Study 4 (SCA10022) and Study 5 (SCA30924). In communication with GlaxoSmithKline, we realized that Study 4 (SCA100222) should actually be SCA100223 which was an acute bipolar depression study. We excluded Study 2 (GW603/SCAA2010) due to different dosing scheme and different length of the treatment phase.

We therefore requested the individual patient-level data from 4 studies from GlaxoSmithKline which included data on:

- `Subject` as patient subject deidentified ID,
- `Age` as patient's age,
- `Sex` as patient's sex,
- `MADRS0` as baseline Montgomery-Asberg Depression Rating Scale,
- `MADRS1` as the final Montgomery-Asberg Depression Rating Scale,
- `HAMD0` as the baseline Hamilton Rating Scale for Depression,
- `HAMD1` as the final Hamilton Rating Scale for Depression,
- `Study` as the indicator of 4 studies and
- `TRT` as the treatment of lamotrigine vs placebo.

Readers interested in analyzing these data or reproducing the results in this chapter should request the individual patient-level data from the company.

We obtained (continuous) data for `MADRS` and `HAMD` and analyzed these data using continuous measures - which is different from Geddes et al. (2009) where numbers of events were aggregated and reported.

The data can be loaded into R and we analyze the difference between the final to baseline as defined as:

```
> # Make the difference between final to baseline
> dat$dMADRS = dat$MADRS1-dat$MADRS0
> dat$dHAMD  = dat$HAMD1-dat$HAMD0
```

There are some missing values in the final `MADRS1` and `HAMD1` and we remove them to consider the complete data as follows:

```
> # Remove missing values
> dat = dat[complete.cases(dat),]
```

We can check our data with the data reported in Table 1 from Geddes et al. (2009). For the Age, the means and standard deviations can be calculated as:

```
> # Calculate the mean
> tapply(dat$Age,dat[,c("TRT","Study")],mean)

     Study
TRT   SCA100223 SCA30924 SCA40910 SCAB2001
  LTG      38.1     40.4     37.6     42.2
  PBO      36.8     38.1     37.2     42.4

> # Calculate the SD
> tapply(dat$Age,dat[,c("TRT","Study")],sd)

     Study
TRT   SCA100223 SCA30924 SCA40910 SCAB2001
  LTG      11.5     12.4     12.7     11.5
  PBO      11.9     12.0     11.5     12.8
```

We can see that the values of these means and SDs by treatment from these four studies are quite similar, but not exactly the same. To further verify the data, we can look into the number of participants with the studies reported in Geddes et al. (2009). The number of patients for each sex by treatment and study can be calculated as follows:

```
> # The number of females
> nF= xtabs(~TRT+Study, dat[dat$Sex=="F",])
> nF

     Study
TRT   SCA100223 SCA30924 SCA40910 SCAB2001
  LTG        70       70       73       35
  PBO        68       65       62       39

> # The number of males
> nM= xtabs(~TRT+Study, dat[dat$Sex=="M",])
```

```
> # The percentage of females
> pctF = nF/(nF+nM)
> pctF

     Study
TRT   SCA100223 SCA30924 SCA40910 SCAB2001
  LTG     0.642    0.556    0.575    0.556
  PBO     0.642    0.533    0.521    0.600
```

Comparing these numbers from this calculation with the values from Table 1 in Geddes et al. (2009), we can see that there are a few minor differences: 1) there are 68 (not 69) female participants in Study SCA10023 for placebo, 2) there are 70 and 65 (not 69 and 66) females for Study SCA30924 from lamotrigine and placebo, and 3) there are 73 (not 74) females for Study SCA40910 from lamotrigine. These differences may be the result of the two analyses using different methods for handling missing data. We will proceed with the data for the comparison between IPD and MA.

8.2 Treatment Comparison for Changes in HAMD

8.2.1 IPD Analysis

8.2.1.1 IPD Analysis by Each Study

Before we analyze the data, we can make distribution plots to investigate the treatment differences graphically. The following R code chunk can be used for this purpose and produces Figure 8.1:

```
> # Load the ``lattice" library
> library(lattice)
> # call boxplot
> print(bwplot(dHAMD~TRT|Study, dat, xlab="Treatment",
 ylab="Changes in HAMD", strip=strip.custom(bg="white")))
```

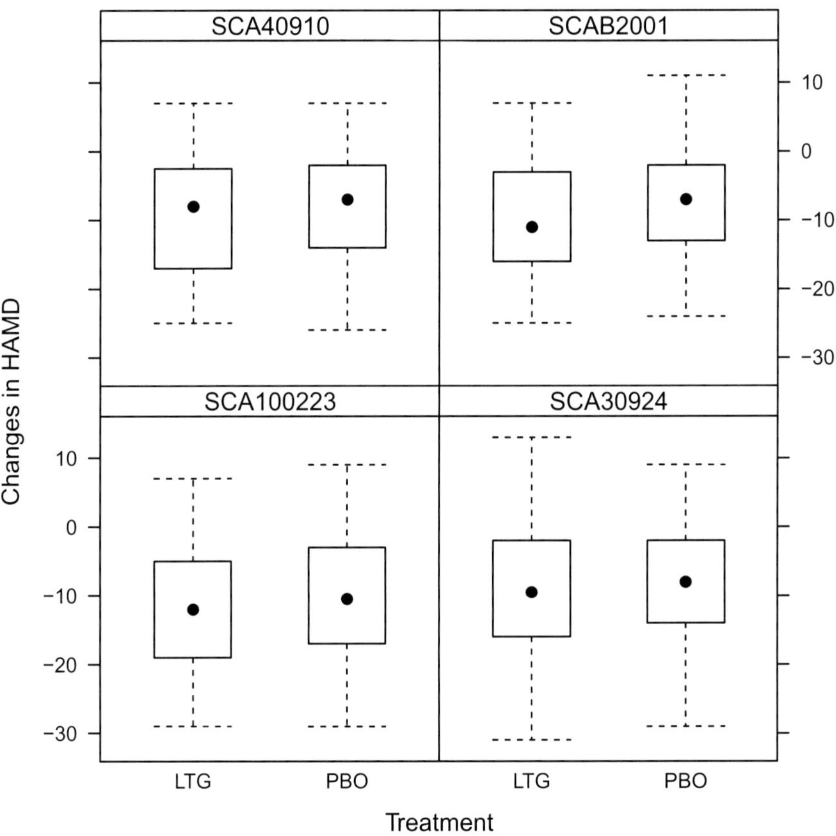

FIGURE 8.1: Boxplot by Treatment for Four Studies

Figure 8.1 illustrates the boxplot for the changes in HAMD by treatment for the four studies. It can be seen that the distributions heavily overlap indicating no statistically significant difference.

This nonsignificance can be statistically tested using the linear model for each study. The analysis for the first data can be implemented by the following R code chunk:

```
> # Test for "SCA100223"
> mStudy1 = lm(dHAMD~TRT, dat[dat$Study==levels(dat$Study)[1],])
> summary(mStudy1)

Call:
lm(formula=dHAMD~TRT,data=dat[dat$Study==levels(dat$Study)[1],])

Residuals:
    Min      1Q  Median      3Q     Max
-19.255  -7.255  -0.459   6.745  18.745

Coefficients:
            Estimate Std. Error t value Pr(>|t|)
(Intercept)  -11.541      0.831  -13.89   <2e-16 ***
TRTPBO         1.796      1.183    1.52     0.13
---
Signif. codes:  0 `***' 0.001 `**' 0.01 `*' 0.05 `.' 0.1 ` ' 1

Residual standard error: 8.67 on 213 degrees of freedom
Multiple R-squared: 0.0107,       Adjusted R-squared: 0.00606
F-statistic:  2.3 on 1 and 213 DF,  p-value: 0.131
```

It can be seen that the associated p-value is 0.131 which indicates a statistically insignificant difference between Lamotrigine and placebo in study SCA100223.

Similarly, the analyses for other three studies can be performed as follows:

```
> # Test for Study "SCA30924"
> mStudy2 = lm(dHAMD~TRT, dat[dat$Study==levels(dat$Study)[2],])
> summary(mStudy2)

Call:
lm(formula=dHAMD~TRT,data=dat[dat$Study==levels(dat$Study)[2],])

Residuals:
    Min      1Q  Median      3Q     Max
-21.746  -6.512   0.566   7.254  22.254

Coefficients:
            Estimate Std. Error t value Pr(>|t|)
(Intercept)   -9.254      0.749  -12.36   <2e-16 ***
TRTPBO         0.688      1.068    0.64     0.52
---
Signif. codes:  0 `***' 0.001 `**' 0.01 `*' 0.05 `.' 0.1 ` ' 1

Residual standard error: 8.41 on 246 degrees of freedom
Multiple R-squared: 0.00169,       Adjusted R-squared: -0.00237
F-statistic: 0.416 on 1 and 246 DF,  p-value: 0.52


> # Test for Study "SCA40910"
> mStudy3 = lm(dHAMD~TRT, dat[dat$Study==levels(dat$Study)[3],])
> summary(mStudy3)

Call:
lm(formula=dHAMD~TRT,data=dat[dat$Study==levels(dat$Study)[3],])

Residuals:
   Min     1Q Median     3Q    Max
-17.35  -6.35   1.41   6.65  16.17

Coefficients:
            Estimate Std. Error t value Pr(>|t|)
```

```
(Intercept)   -9.173      0.726   -12.6   <2e-16 ***
TRTPBO         0.526      1.044     0.5     0.61
---
Signif. codes:  0 `***' 0.001 `**' 0.01 `*' 0.05 `.' 0.1 ` ' 1

Residual standard error: 8.19 on 244 degrees of freedom
Multiple R-squared: 0.00104,        Adjusted R-squared: -0.00305
F-statistic: 0.254 on 1 and 244 DF,  p-value: 0.615

> # Test for Study "SCAB2001"
> mStudy4 = lm(dHAMD~TRT, dat[dat$Study==levels(dat$Study)[4],])
> summary(mStudy4)

Call:
lm(formula=dHAMD~TRT,data=dat[dat$Study==levels(dat$Study)[4],])

Residuals:
    Min      1Q  Median      3Q     Max
-16.185  -5.261   0.162   6.585  18.815

Coefficients:
            Estimate Std. Error t value Pr(>|t|)
(Intercept)   -10.51       1.01   -10.4   <2e-16 ***
TRTPBO          2.69       1.41     1.9    0.059 .
---
Signif. codes:  0 `***' 0.001 `**' 0.01 `*' 0.05 `.' 0.1 ` ' 1

Residual standard error: 8 on 126 degrees of freedom
Multiple R-squared: 0.028,        Adjusted R-squared: 0.0203
F-statistic: 3.63 on 1 and 126 DF,  p-value: 0.0592
```

The associated p-values are 0.52 for study `SCA30924`, 0.615 for study `SCA40910` and 0.059 for study `SCAB2001`, respectively. None are statistically significant at the 0.05 level, indicating that Lamotrigine is not statistically more effective than the placebo in treating bipolar depression if the data are analyzed by study.

8.2.1.2 IPD Analysis with Pooled Data

For the IPD analysis, we can pool the four studies together to test treatment and study interaction effects as follows:

```
> # Model the interaction
> m1 = lm(dHAMD~TRT*Study, dat)
> # Print the ANOVA result
> anova(m1)

Analysis of Variance Table

Response: dHAMD
           Df Sum Sq Mean Sq F value Pr(>F)
TRT         1    316   315.5    4.52  0.034 *
Study       3    465   154.9    2.22  0.084 .
TRT:Study   3    134    44.8    0.64  0.588
Residuals 829  57820    69.7
---
Signif. codes:  0 `***' 0.001 `**' 0.01 `*' 0.05 `.' 0.1 ` ' 1
```

We can see that the treatment is now statistically significant (p-value $=0.0337$) and the interaction is not statistically significant (p-value $= 0.5883$). We then reduce the model by excluding the interaction term - which is to regard study as a block. In this situation, the test for treatment effect can be carried out using the following R code chunk:

```
> # Model the main effect
> m2 = lm(dHAMD~TRT+Study, dat)
> # Print the ANOVA result
> anova(m2)

Analysis of Variance Table

Response: dHAMD
           Df Sum Sq Mean Sq F value Pr(>F)
TRT         1    316   315.5    4.53  0.034 *
Study       3    465   154.9    2.22  0.084 .
```

```
Residuals 832  57954    69.7
---
Signif. codes:  0 `***' 0.001 `**' 0.01 `*' 0.05 `.' 0.1 ` ' 1
```

Again the treatment effect is statistically significant (p-value =0.0336) and there is no statistically significant difference among the 4 studies (p-value = 0.0839). A Tukey multiple comparison procedure can be further performed to confirm this conclusion which can be done as follows:

```
> TukeyHSD(aov(dHAMD~TRT+Study, dat))

  Tukey multiple comparisons of means
    95% family-wise confidence level


Fit: aov(formula = dHAMD ~ TRT + Study, data = dat)


$TRT
        diff    lwr  upr p adj
PBO-LTG 1.23 0.0955 2.36 0.034


$Study
                       diff    lwr  upr p adj
SCA30924-SCA100223  1.74183 -0.260 3.74 0.114
SCA40910-SCA100223  1.74852 -0.257 3.75 0.112
SCAB2001-SCA100223  1.49703 -0.902 3.90 0.375
SCA40910-SCA30924   0.00669 -1.927 1.94 1.000
SCAB2001-SCA30924  -0.24480 -2.583 2.09 0.993
SCAB2001-SCA40910  -0.25149 -2.593 2.09 0.993
```

In summary, when data are pooled from the four studies, the treatment effect is now statistically significant in contrast to nonsignificance in the IPD analysis for each study in Section 8.2.1.1. This is expected since when data are pooled, the statistical power is usually increased.

8.2.1.3 IPD Analysis Incorporating Covariates

It is well known that the major advantage in IPD analysis is the capacity to incorporate covariates. For this data, we have individual patient level data from Age and Sex. We can then incorporate these covariates into the linear model. We model the interactions between TRT and Study as follows:

```
> # Full model
> mAllStudy1 = lm(dHAMD~(Age+Sex)*TRT*Study, dat)
> # Print the ANOVA
> anova(mAllStudy1)

Analysis of Variance Table

Response: dHAMD
               Df Sum Sq Mean Sq F value Pr(>F)
Age             1    160     160    2.30  0.130
Sex             1     10      10    0.14  0.706
TRT             1    334     334    4.81  0.029 *
Study           3    435     145    2.08  0.101
Age:TRT         1      8       8    0.11  0.737
Sex:TRT         1     22      22    0.31  0.578
Age:Study       3    299     100    1.43  0.231
Sex:Study       3    310     103    1.48  0.217
TRT:Study       3    116      39    0.56  0.643
Age:TRT:Study   3    240      80    1.15  0.327
Sex:TRT:Study   3    227      76    1.09  0.353
Residuals     813  56572      70
---
Signif. codes:  0 `***' 0.001 `**' 0.01 `*' 0.05 `.' 0.1 ` ' 1
```

From the results, we can see that all 2-way and 3-way interactions are statistically nonsignificant. We reduce the model to the main effects as follows:

```
> # Fit the main effect model
> mAllStudy2 = lm(dHAMD~TRT+Study+Age+Sex, dat)
> # Print the ANOVA
> anova(mAllStudy2)

Analysis of Variance Table
```

```
Response: dHAMD
           Df Sum Sq Mean Sq F value Pr(>F)
TRT         1    316   315.5    4.53  0.034 *
Study       3    465   154.9    2.23  0.084 .
Age         1    158   157.7    2.27  0.133
Sex         1      1     1.3    0.02  0.891
Residuals 830  57795    69.6
---
Signif. codes:  0 `***' 0.001 `**' 0.01 `*' 0.05 `.' 0.1 ` ' 1
```

The `Sex` and `Age` are not statistically significant which indicates that we can further reduce the model to the main effects of `TRT` and `Study` which is the model `m2` above.

8.2.1.4 Summary of IPD Analysis

In summary, when the data from each study are analyzed separately, lamotrigine is not statistically more effective than the placebo. When the data from all four studies are combined as a pooled IPD analysis, lamotrigine is statistically more effective than the placebo. Furthermore there is no statistically significant difference among the studies, indicating no statistically significant heterogeneity among the four studies. In addition, `Age` and `Sex` are not significant covariates.

8.2.2 Meta-Analysis

To carry out the meta-analysis, we make use of R library `metafor`. We `aggregate` the individual patient-level data into study-level summaries as follows:

```
> # Get the number of observations
> nHAMD = aggregate(dat$dHAMD,
         list(Study=dat$Study,TRT = dat$TRT), length)
> nHAMD

      Study TRT   x
1 SCA100223 LTG 109
2  SCA30924 LTG 126
```

```
3  SCA40910 LTG 127
4  SCAB2001 LTG  63
5 SCA100223 PBO 106
6  SCA30924 PBO 122
7  SCA40910 PBO 119
8  SCAB2001 PBO  65

> # Calculate the means
> mHAMD = aggregate(dat$dHAMD,
        list(Study=dat$Study,TRT = dat$TRT), mean)
> mHAMD

      Study TRT      x
1 SCA100223 LTG -11.54
2  SCA30924 LTG  -9.25
3  SCA40910 LTG  -9.17
4  SCAB2001 LTG -10.51
5 SCA100223 PBO  -9.75
6  SCA30924 PBO  -8.57
7  SCA40910 PBO  -8.65
8  SCAB2001 PBO  -7.82

> # Calculate the SD
> sdHAMD = aggregate(dat$dHAMD,
        list(Study=dat$Study,TRT = dat$TRT), sd)
> sdHAMD

      Study TRT    x
1 SCA100223 LTG 8.75
2  SCA30924 LTG 8.11
3  SCA40910 LTG 8.42
4  SCAB2001 LTG 8.11
5 SCA100223 PBO 8.60
6  SCA30924 PBO 8.70
7  SCA40910 PBO 7.93
8  SCAB2001 PBO 7.89
```

With these study-level summaries, we first calculate the effect-size (ES). Since HAMD is reported with the same unit from all studies we use the simple mean difference (MD) which can be specified in `measure="MD"`. The R code chunk is as follows:

```
> # Load the library
> library(metafor)
> # Calculate the effect size
> esHAMD = escalc(measure="MD",
         n1i= nHAMD$x[nHAMD$TRT=="LTG"],
         n2i= nHAMD$x[nHAMD$TRT=="PBO"],
         m1i= mHAMD$x[mHAMD$TRT=="LTG"],
         m2i= mHAMD$x[mHAMD$TRT=="PBO"],
         sd1i= sdHAMD$x[sdHAMD$TRT=="LTG"],
         sd2i= sdHAMD$x[sdHAMD$TRT=="PBO"], append=T)
> # Use the study name as row name
> rownames(esHAMD) = nHAMD$Study[nHAMD$TRT=="LTG"]
> # Print the calculated ESs and SDs
> esHAMD
```

```
              yi   vi
SCA100223 -1.796 1.40
SCA30924  -0.688 1.14
SCA40910  -0.526 1.09
SCAB2001  -2.693 2.00
```

Based on these ESs, we can calculate the p-values associated with each study as follows:

```
> # Calculate the z-values
> z = esHAMD$yi/sqrt(esHAMD$vi)
> # Calculate the p-values
> pval = 2*(1-pnorm(abs(z)))
> # Print the p-values
> pval
```

```
[1] 0.129 0.520 0.614 0.057
attr(,"measure")
[1] "MD"
```

We can see from these studywise p-values that none of the four studies demonstrated statistical significance for lamotrigine as compared to placebo - which is similar to the IPD analysis of each study.

Now we can come to perform the meta-analysis. We fit the fixed-effects meta-model and the series of random-effects meta-models to compare the results.

The fixed-effects meta-analysis can be carried out by the following R code chunk:

```
> # The fixed-effects meta-analysis
> metaHAMD.MD.FE = rma(yi,vi,measure="MD",
                  method="FE", data=esHAMD)
> metaHAMD.MD.FE

Fixed-Effects Model (k = 4)

Test for Heterogeneity:
Q(df = 3) = 2.0102, p-val = 0.5703

Model Results:
estimate       se     zval     pval    ci.lb    ci.ub
 -1.2345   0.5764  -2.1416   0.0322  -2.3642  -0.1047 *
---
Signif. codes:  0 `***' 0.001 `**' 0.01 `*' 0.05 `.' 0.1 ` ' 1
```

It can be seen that the associated p-value is 0.032 for the mean difference of -1.234 indicating statistically significant treatment effect.

We fit a series of random-effects models using different estimation methods to estimate the between-study heterogeneity. These model-fittings can be easily implemented as follows:

```
> # The random-effects meta-analysis with "DL"
```

```
> metaHAMD.MD.DL = rma(yi,vi,measure="MD",
                 method="DL", data=esHAMD)
> metaHAMD.MD.DL

Random-Effects Model (k = 4; tau^2 estimator: DL)

tau^2 (estimate of total amount of heterogeneity): 0
tau (sqrt of the estimate of total heterogeneity): 0
I^2 (% of total variability due to heterogeneity): 0.00%
H^2 (total variability / sampling variability):    1.00

Test for Heterogeneity:
Q(df = 3) = 2.0102, p-val = 0.5703

Model Results:
estimate      se     zval     pval    ci.lb    ci.ub
 -1.2345  0.5764  -2.1416   0.0322  -2.3642  -0.1047 *
---
Signif. codes:  0 `***' 0.001 `**' 0.01 `*' 0.05 `.' 0.1 ` ' 1


> # The random-effects meta-analysis with "HS"
> metaHAMD.MD.HS = rma(yi,vi,measure="MD",
                 method="HS", data=esHAMD)
> metaHAMD.MD.HS

Random-Effects Model (k = 4; tau^2 estimator: HS)

tau^2 (estimate of total amount of heterogeneity): 0
tau (sqrt of the estimate of total heterogeneity): 0
I^2 (% of total variability due to heterogeneity): 0.00%
H^2 (total variability / sampling variability):    1.00

Test for Heterogeneity:
Q(df = 3) = 2.0102, p-val = 0.5703
```

```
Model Results:
estimate       se      zval     pval    ci.lb    ci.ub
 -1.2345   0.5764  -2.1416   0.0322  -2.3642  -0.1047 *
---
Signif. codes:  0 `***' 0.001 `**' 0.01 `*' 0.05 `.' 0.1 ` ' 1


> # The random-effects meta-analysis with "HE"
> metaHAMD.MD.HE = rma(yi,vi,measure="MD",
                  method="HE", data=esHAMD)
> metaHAMD.MD.HE

Random-Effects Model (k = 4; tau^2 estimator: HE)

tau^2 (estimate of total amount of heterogeneity): 0
tau (sqrt of the estimate of total heterogeneity): 0
I^2 (% of total variability due to heterogeneity): 0.00%
H^2 (total variability / sampling variability):    1.00

Test for Heterogeneity:
Q(df = 3) = 2.0102, p-val = 0.5703

Model Results:
estimate       se      zval     pval    ci.lb    ci.ub
 -1.2345   0.5764  -2.1416   0.0322  -2.3642  -0.1047 *
---
Signif. codes:  0 `***' 0.001 `**' 0.01 `*' 0.05 `.' 0.1 ` ' 1


> # The random-effects meta-analysis with "SJ"
> metaHAMD.MD.SJ = rma(yi,vi,measure="MD",
                  method="SJ", data=esHAMD)
> metaHAMD.MD.SJ

Random-Effects Model (k = 4; tau^2 estimator: SJ)

tau^2 (estimate of total amount of heterogeneity): 0.3428
```

```
tau (sqrt of the estimate of total heterogeneity): 0.5855
I^2 (% of total variability due to heterogeneity): 20.24%
H^2 (total variability / sampling variability):    1.25

Test for Heterogeneity:
Q(df = 3) = 2.0102, p-val = 0.5703

Model Results:
estimate       se     zval     pval    ci.lb    ci.ub
 -1.2686   0.6491  -1.9545   0.0506  -2.5408   0.0036 .
---
Signif. codes:  0 `***' 0.001 `**' 0.01 `*' 0.05 `.' 0.1 ` ' 1


> # The random-effects meta-analysis with "ML"
> metaHAMD.MD.ML = rma(yi,vi,measure="MD",
                  method="ML", data=esHAMD)
> metaHAMD.MD.ML

Random-Effects Model (k = 4; tau^2 estimator: ML)

tau^2(estimate of total amount of heterogeneity): 0(SE=0.92)
tau (sqrt of the estimate of total heterogeneity): 0
I^2 (% of total variability due to heterogeneity): 0.00%
H^2 (total variability / sampling variability):    1.00

Test for Heterogeneity:
Q(df = 3) = 2.0102, p-val = 0.5703

Model Results:
estimate       se     zval     pval    ci.lb    ci.ub
 -1.2345   0.5764  -2.1416   0.0322  -2.3642  -0.1047 *
---
Signif. codes:  0 `***' 0.001 `**' 0.01 `*' 0.05 `.' 0.1 ` ' 1


> # The random-effects meta-analysis with "REML"
```

```
> metaHAMD.MD.REML = rma(yi,vi,measure="MD",
               method="REML", data=esHAMD)
> metaHAMD.MD.REML

Random-Effects Model (k = 4; tau^2 estimator: REML)

tau^2(estimate of total amount of heterogeneity): 0(SE=1.08)
tau (sqrt of the estimate of total heterogeneity): 0
I^2 (% of total variability due to heterogeneity): 0.00%
H^2 (total variability / sampling variability):    1.00

Test for Heterogeneity:
Q(df = 3) = 2.0102, p-val = 0.5703

Model Results:
estimate       se     zval     pval    ci.lb    ci.ub
 -1.2345   0.5764  -2.1416   0.0322  -2.3642  -0.1047 *
---
Signif. codes:  0 `***' 0.001 `**' 0.01 `*' 0.05 `.' 0.1 ` ' 1


> # The random-effects meta-analysis with "EB"
> metaHAMD.MD.EB = rma(yi,vi,measure="MD",
               method="EB", data=esHAMD)
> metaHAMD.MD.EB

Random-Effects Model (k = 4; tau^2 estimator: EB)

tau^2 (estimate of total amount of heterogeneity): 0
tau (sqrt of the estimate of total heterogeneity): 0
I^2 (% of total variability due to heterogeneity): 0.00%
H^2 (total variability / sampling variability):    1.00

Test for Heterogeneity:
Q(df = 3) = 2.0102, p-val = 0.5703
```

```
Model Results:

estimate       se      zval      pval     ci.lb     ci.ub
 -1.2345   0.5764   -2.1416   0.0322   -2.3642   -0.1047 *

---

Signif. codes:  0 `***' 0.001 `**' 0.01 `*' 0.05 `.' 0.1 ` ' 1
```

From the above model-fittings, all `Test of Heterogeneity` are not statistically significant, and the treatment effect is significant with p-value of 0.0322 from all models which yields the same conclusion as the IPD pooled data analysis. The conclusion can be illustrated using the forest plot from `DL` with a simple R code `forest(metaHAMD.MD.DL, slab=rownames(esHAMD))` which is shown in Figure 8.2.

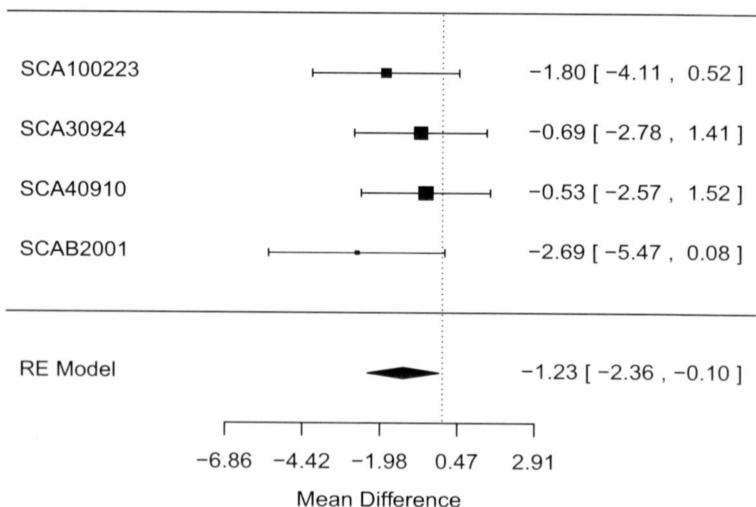

FIGURE 8.2: Forest Plot for HAMD

8.3 Treatment Comparison for Changes in MADRS

We follow the same procedure as in the last section to analyze the MADRS without further explanations.

8.3.1 IPD Analysis

We first test the significance using data from each study as follows:

```
> # Test for Study "SCA100223"
> mStudy1 = lm(dMADRS~TRT, dat[dat$Study==levels(dat$Study)[1],])
> summary(mStudy1)

Call:
lm(formula=dMADRS~TRT,data=dat[dat$Study==levels(dat$Study)[1],])


Residuals:
   Min     1Q Median     3Q    Max
-20.35  -9.24  -1.35  10.21  26.65


Coefficients:
            Estimate Std. Error t value Pr(>|t|)
(Intercept)  -13.651      1.052  -12.98   <2e-16 ***
TRTPBO         0.887      1.498    0.59     0.55
---
Signif. codes:  0 `***' 0.001 `**' 0.01 `*' 0.05 `.' 0.1 ` ' 1

Residual standard error: 11 on 213 degrees of freedom
Multiple R-squared: 0.00164,       Adjusted R-squared: -0.00304
F-statistic: 0.351 on 1 and 213 DF,  p-value: 0.554


> # Test for Study "SCA30924"
> mStudy2 = lm(dMADRS~TRT, dat[dat$Study==levels(dat$Study)[2],])
> summary(mStudy2)
```

```
Call:
lm(formula=dMADRS~TRT,data=dat[dat$Study==levels(dat$Study)[2],])

Residuals:
   Min     1Q Median     3Q    Max 
-24.98  -8.22   1.07   9.07  26.02 

Coefficients:
            Estimate Std. Error t value Pr(>|t|)    
(Intercept)  -12.016      0.989  -12.15   <2e-16 ***
TRTPBO         0.950      1.410    0.67      0.5    
---
Signif. codes:  0 `***' 0.001 `**' 0.01 `*' 0.05 `.' 0.1 ` ' 1

Residual standard error: 11.1 on 246 degrees of freedom
Multiple R-squared: 0.00184,	Adjusted R-squared: -0.00222 
F-statistic: 0.454 on 1 and 246 DF,  p-value: 0.501 


> # Test for Study "SCA40910"
> mStudy3 = lm(dMADRS~TRT, dat[dat$Study==levels(dat$Study)[3],])
> summary(mStudy3)

Call:
lm(formula=dMADRS~TRT,data=dat[dat$Study==levels(dat$Study)[3],])

Residuals:
    Min      1Q  Median      3Q     Max 
-27.975  -8.940   0.595   9.130  31.165 

Coefficients:
            Estimate Std. Error t value Pr(>|t|)    
(Intercept)   -12.17       1.04  -11.71   <2e-16 ***
TRTPBO          1.14       1.49    0.76     0.45    
---
Signif. codes:  0 `***' 0.001 `**' 0.01 `*' 0.05 `.' 0.1 ` ' 1
```

```
Residual standard error: 11.7 on 244 degrees of freedom
Multiple R-squared: 0.00238,       Adjusted R-squared: -0.00171
F-statistic: 0.583 on 1 and 244 DF,  p-value: 0.446


> # Test for Study "SCAB2001"
> mStudy4 = lm(dMADRS~TRT, dat[dat$Study==levels(dat$Study)[4],])
> summary(mStudy4)

Call:
lm(formula=dMADRS~TRT,data=dat[dat$Study==levels(dat$Study)[4],])

Residuals:
    Min      1Q  Median      3Q     Max
-23.215  -8.851  -0.473   8.270  23.270

Coefficients:
            Estimate Std. Error t value Pr(>|t|)
(Intercept)   -13.27       1.38   -9.63   <2e-16 ***
TRTPBO          5.49       1.93    2.84   0.0053 **
---
Signif. codes:  0 `***' 0.001 `**' 0.01 `*' 0.05 `.' 0.1 ` ' 1

Residual standard error: 10.9 on 126 degrees of freedom
Multiple R-squared: 0.06,       Adjusted R-squared: 0.0526
F-statistic: 8.05 on 1 and 126 DF,  p-value: 0.00531
```

We can see that when data are analyzed for each study, there is no statistical significance for the first three studies (i.e. `SCA100223`, `SCA30924` and `SCA40910`); however, there is statistical significance from the fourth study (i.e. `SCAB2001`).

We pool the four studies together to test treatment and study interaction as follows:

```
> # Model the interaction
> m1 = lm(dMADRS~TRT*Study, dat)
> # Print the ANOVA result
> anova(m1)

Analysis of Variance Table

Response: dMADRS
           Df Sum Sq Mean Sq F value Pr(>F)
TRT         1    599     599    4.75   0.03 *
Study       3    668     223    1.77   0.15
TRT:Study   3    548     183    1.45   0.23
Residuals 829 104515     126
---
Signif. codes:  0 `***' 0.001 `**' 0.01 `*' 0.05 `.' 0.1 ` ' 1
```

We can see that the treatment effect is now statistically significant (p-value =0.02952) and the interaction is not statistically significant (p-value = 0.22727). We then exclude the interaction and test the main effect as follows:

```
> # Model the main effect
> m2 = lm(dMADRS~TRT+Study, dat)
> # Print the ANOVA result
> anova(m2)

Analysis of Variance Table

Response: dMADRS
           Df Sum Sq Mean Sq F value Pr(>F)
TRT         1    599     599    4.75   0.03 *
Study       3    668     223    1.76   0.15
Residuals 832 105063     126
---
Signif. codes:  0 `***' 0.001 `**' 0.01 `*' 0.05 `.' 0.1 ` ' 1
```

Again the treatment effect is statistically significant (p-value =0.02965) and there is no statistically significant difference among the four studies (p-

value = 0.1525). A Tukey multiple comparison procedure can be further performed to confirm this conclusion which can be done as follows:

```
> TukeyHSD(aov(dMADRS~TRT+Study, dat))

  Tukey multiple comparisons of means
    95% family-wise confidence level

Fit: aov(formula = dMADRS ~ TRT + Study, data = dat)

$TRT
        diff   lwr  upr p adj
PBO-LTG 1.69 0.168 3.22  0.03

$Study
                        diff    lwr  upr p adj
SCA30924-SCA100223  1.6674 -1.028 4.36 0.384
SCA40910-SCA100223  1.6158 -1.085 4.32 0.414
SCAB2001-SCA100223  2.7045 -0.525 5.93 0.137
SCA40910-SCA30924  -0.0516 -2.655 2.55 1.000
SCAB2001-SCA30924   1.0371 -2.111 4.19 0.831
SCAB2001-SCA40910   1.0887 -2.064 4.24 0.811
```

Similarly, we can incorporate the covariates `Age` and `Sex` to test the `TRT` and `Study` significance as follows:

```
> # Full model
> mAllStudy1 = lm(dMADRS~(Age+Sex)*TRT*Study, dat)
> # Print the ANOVA
> anova(mAllStudy1)

Analysis of Variance Table

Response: dMADRS
               Df Sum Sq Mean Sq F value Pr(>F)
Age             1    173     173    1.37  0.242
Sex             1     55      55    0.44  0.510
```

```
TRT              1    623     623    4.93  0.027 *
Study            3    584     195    1.54  0.202
Age:TRT          1     26      26    0.21  0.650
Sex:TRT          1      0       0    0.00  0.993
Age:Study        3    578     193    1.53  0.206
Sex:Study        3    285      95    0.75  0.521
TRT:Study        3    499     166    1.32  0.267
Age:TRT:Study    3    159      53    0.42  0.739
Sex:TRT:Study    3    759     253    2.01  0.112
Residuals      813 102589     126
---
Signif. codes:  0 `***' 0.001 `**' 0.01 `*' 0.05 `.' 0.1 ` ' 1
```

Since there is no statistical significance for all the 2-way and 3-way interactions, we fit the main effect model as follows:

```
> # Fit the main effect model
> mAllStudy2 = lm(dMADRS~TRT+Study+Age+Sex, dat)
> # Print the ANOVA
> anova(mAllStudy2)

Analysis of Variance Table

Response: dMADRS
           Df Sum Sq Mean Sq F value Pr(>F)
TRT         1    599     599    4.74   0.03 *
Study       3    668     223    1.76   0.15
Age         1    137     137    1.08   0.30
Sex         1     31      31    0.24   0.62
Residuals 830 104896     126
---
Signif. codes:  0 `***' 0.001 `**' 0.01 `*' 0.05 `.' 0.1 ` ' 1
```

Again, `Sex` and `Age` are not statistically significant which indicates that we can further reduce the model to the main effects `TRT` and `Study` which is the model `m2` above.

8.3.2 Meta-Analysis

Similarly, we first aggregate the individual patient-level data into study-level summaries as follows:

```
> # Get the number of observations
> nMADRS = aggregate(dat$dMADRS,
    list(Study=dat$Study,TRT = dat$TRT), length)
> nMADRS

      Study TRT   x
1 SCA100223 LTG 109
2  SCA30924 LTG 126
3  SCA40910 LTG 127
4  SCAB2001 LTG  63
5 SCA100223 PBO 106
6  SCA30924 PBO 122
7  SCA40910 PBO 119
8  SCAB2001 PBO  65

> # Calculate the means
> mMADRS = aggregate(dat$dMADRS,
    list(Study=dat$Study,TRT = dat$TRT), mean)
> mMADRS

      Study TRT      x
1 SCA100223 LTG -13.65
2  SCA30924 LTG -12.02
3  SCA40910 LTG -12.17
4  SCAB2001 LTG -13.27
5 SCA100223 PBO -12.76
6  SCA30924 PBO -11.07
7  SCA40910 PBO -11.03
8  SCAB2001 PBO  -7.78

> # Calculate the SD
> sdMADRS = aggregate(dat$dMADRS,
    list(Study=dat$Study,TRT = dat$TRT), sd)
> sdMADRS
```

```
      Study TRT    x
1 SCA100223 LTG 11.1
2  SCA30924 LTG 10.8
3  SCA40910 LTG 11.8
4  SCAB2001 LTG 11.5
5 SCA100223 PBO 10.9
6  SCA30924 PBO 11.4
7  SCA40910 PBO 11.6
8  SCAB2001 PBO 10.4
```

We then calculate the effect-size (ES) using the simple mean difference (MD) with following R code chunk:

```
> # Calculate the effect size
> esMADRS = escalc(measure="MD",
         n1i= nMADRS$x[nMADRS$TRT=="LTG"],
         n2i= nMADRS$x[nMADRS$TRT=="PBO"],
         m1i= mMADRS$x[mMADRS$TRT=="LTG"],
         m2i= mMADRS$x[mMADRS$TRT=="PBO"],
         sd1i= sdMADRS$x[sdMADRS$TRT=="LTG"],
         sd2i= sdMADRS$x[sdMADRS$TRT=="PBO"], append=T)
> # Use the study name as row name
> rownames(esMADRS) = nMADRS$Study[nMADRS$TRT=="LTG"]
> # Print the data
> esMADRS

              yi   vi
SCA100223 -0.887 2.24
SCA30924  -0.950 1.99
SCA40910  -1.140 2.23
SCAB2001  -5.485 3.75
```

Based on these ESs, we calculate the p-values associated with each study as follows:

```
> # Calculate the z-values
> z = esMADRS$yi/sqrt(esMADRS$vi)
```

```
> # Calculate the p-values
> pval = 2*(1-pnorm(abs(z)))
> # Print the p-values
> pval

[1] 0.55350 0.50084 0.44494 0.00462
attr(,"measure")
[1] "MD"
```

Again from these p-values, the treatment effect is not statistically significant for first three studies. For the meta-analysis, we fit the fixed-effects meta-model and the series of random-effects meta-model, to compare the results, which can be easily implemented in R as follows:

```
> # The fixed-effects meta-analysis
> metaMADRS.MD.FE = rma(yi,vi,measure="MD",
                          method="FE", data=esMADRS)
> metaMADRS.MD.FE

Fixed-Effects Model (k = 4)


Test for Heterogeneity:
Q(df = 3) = 4.5375, p-val = 0.2090


Model Results:
estimate       se     zval     pval    ci.lb    ci.ub
 -1.7116   0.7754  -2.2074   0.0273  -3.2313  -0.1919 *
---
Signif. codes:  0 `***' 0.001 `**' 0.01 `*' 0.05 `.' 0.1 ` ' 1


> # The random-effects meta-analysis with "DL"
> metaMADRS.MD.DL = rma(yi,vi,measure="MD",
                          method="DL", data=esMADRS)
> metaMADRS.MD.DL

Random-Effects Model (k = 4; tau^2 estimator: DL)
```

```
tau^2 (estimate of total amount of heterogeneity): 1.2516
tau (sqrt of the estimate of total heterogeneity): 1.1187
I^2 (% of total variability due to heterogeneity): 33.88%
H^2 (total variability / sampling variability):    1.51

Test for Heterogeneity:
Q(df = 3) = 4.5375, p-val = 0.2090

Model Results:
estimate       se      zval     pval     ci.lb    ci.ub
 -1.8221   0.9615  -1.8952   0.0581  -3.7066   0.0623.
---
Signif. codes:  0 `***' 0.001 `**' 0.01 `*' 0.05 `.' 0.1 ` ' 1


> # The random-effects meta-analysis with "HS"
> metaMADRS.MD.HS = rma(yi,vi,measure="MD",
                          method="HS", data=esMADRS)
> metaMADRS.MD.HS

Random-Effects Model (k = 4; tau^2 estimator: HS)

tau^2 (estimate of total amount of heterogeneity): 0.3231
tau (sqrt of the estimate of total heterogeneity): 0.5685
I^2 (% of total variability due to heterogeneity): 11.69%
H^2 (total variability / sampling variability):    1.13

Test for Heterogeneity:
Q(df = 3) = 4.5375, p-val = 0.2090

Model Results:
estimate       se      zval     pval     ci.lb    ci.ub
 -1.7474   0.8279  -2.1108   0.0348  -3.3700  -0.1248 *
---
Signif. codes:  0 `***' 0.001 `**' 0.01 `*' 0.05 `.' 0.1 ` ' 1
```

```
> # The random-effects meta-analysis with "HE"
> metaMADRS.MD.HE = rma(yi,vi,measure="MD",
                          method="HE", data=esMADRS)
> metaMADRS.MD.HE

Random-Effects Model (k = 4; tau^2 estimator: HE)

tau^2 (estimate of total amount of heterogeneity): 2.5043
tau (sqrt of the estimate of total heterogeneity): 1.5825
I^2 (% of total variability due to heterogeneity): 50.63%
H^2 (total variability / sampling variability):    2.03

Test for Heterogeneity:
Q(df = 3) = 4.5375, p-val = 0.2090

Model Results:
estimate       se      zval     pval    ci.lb    ci.ub
 -1.8852   1.1151   -1.6906   0.0909  -4.0707   0.3003 .
---
Signif. codes:  0 `***' 0.001 `**' 0.01 `*' 0.05 `.' 0.1 ` ' 1


> # The random-effects meta-analysis with "SJ"
> metaMADRS.MD.SJ = rma(yi,vi,measure="MD",
                          method="SJ", data=esMADRS)
> metaMADRS.MD.SJ

Random-Effects Model (k = 4; tau^2 estimator: SJ)

tau^2 (estimate of total amount of heterogeneity): 2.6871
tau (sqrt of the estimate of total heterogeneity): 1.6392
I^2 (% of total variability due to heterogeneity): 52.39%
H^2 (total variability / sampling variability):    2.10

Test for Heterogeneity:
```

```
Q(df = 3) = 4.5375, p-val = 0.2090

Model Results:
estimate       se      zval      pval    ci.lb     ci.ub
 -1.8922   1.1357  -1.6661   0.0957  -4.1180   0.3337.
---
Signif. codes:  0 `***' 0.001 `**' 0.01 `*' 0.05 `.' 0.1 ` ' 1


> # The random-effects meta-analysis with "ML"
> metaMADRS.MD.ML = rma(yi,vi,measure="MD",
                          method="ML", data=esMADRS)
> metaMADRS.MD.ML

Random-Effects Model (k = 4; tau^2 estimator: ML)

tau^2(estimate of total amount of heterogeneity):0(SE=1.6629)
tau (sqrt of the estimate of total heterogeneity): 0.0010
I^2 (% of total variability due to heterogeneity): 0.00%
H^2 (total variability / sampling variability):    1.00

Test for Heterogeneity:
Q(df = 3) = 4.5375, p-val = 0.2090

Model Results:
estimate       se      zval      pval    ci.lb     ci.ub
 -1.7116   0.7754  -2.2074   0.0273  -3.2313  -0.1919 *
---
Signif. codes:  0 `***' 0.001 `**' 0.01 `*' 0.05 `.' 0.1 ` ' 1


> # The random-effects meta-analysis with "REML"
> metaMADRS.MD.REML = rma(yi,vi,measure="MD",
                          method="REML", data=esMADRS)
> metaMADRS.MD.REML
```

```
Random-Effects Model (k = 4; tau^2 estimator: REML)

tau^2(estimate of total amount of heterogeneity):0.57(SE=2.44)
tau (sqrt of the estimate of total heterogeneity): 0.7595
I^2 (% of total variability due to heterogeneity): 19.11%
H^2 (total variability / sampling variability):    1.24

Test for Heterogeneity:
Q(df = 3) = 4.5375, p-val = 0.2090

Model Results:
estimate       se     zval     pval    ci.lb    ci.ub
 -1.7714   0.8666  -2.0440   0.0409  -3.4699  -0.0729 *
---
Signif. codes:  0 `***' 0.001 `**' 0.01 `*' 0.05 `.' 0.1 ` ' 1



> # The random-effects meta-analysis with "EB"
> metaMADRS.MD.EB = rma(yi,vi,measure="MD",
                          method="EB", data=esMADRS)
> metaMADRS.MD.EB

Random-Effects Model (k = 4; tau^2 estimator: EB)

tau^2 (estimate of total amount of heterogeneity): 1.7121
tau (sqrt of the estimate of total heterogeneity): 1.3085
I^2 (% of total variability due to heterogeneity): 41.21%
H^2 (total variability / sampling variability):    1.70

Test for Heterogeneity:
Q(df = 3) = 4.5375, p-val = 0.2090

Model Results:
estimate       se     zval     pval    ci.lb    ci.ub
 -1.8490   1.0208  -1.8113   0.0701  -3.8497   0.1518 .
```

```
---
Signif. codes:  0 `***' 0.001 `**' 0.01 `*' 0.05 `.' 0.1 ` ' 1
```

The same conclusion can be made that all `Test of Heterogeneity` are not statistically significant, but the treatment effect is statistically significant, which yields the same conclusion as the IPD pooled analysis.

8.4 Summary

In the above analysis, we used the simple mean difference by specifying `measure="MD"`. We also analyzed this data using *standardized mean difference* which can be specified easily by using `measure="SMD"`, and we found the same conclusions.

In summary, when data from each study are analyzed separately, lamotrigine is not statistically more effective than the placebo in `HAMD`. For `MADRS`, there is a statistical significance in study `SCAB2001`, but not for the other three studies of `SCA100223`, `SCA30924` and `SCA40910`. However, when data from all four studies are pooled using the IPD pooled analysis and the meta-analysis, lamotrigine is statistically more effective than the placebo. Furthermore there is no statistically significant difference among the studies indicating that there is no statistically significant heterogeneity among the four studies.

From the analysis, we can see that both the IPD pooled analysis and meta-analysis from the aggregated data yielded similar conclusions. In fact this is true in general as demonstrated in Lin and Zeng (2010) in the setting of fixed-effects model. In this paper, the authors showed theoretically that for all commonly used parametric and semiparametric models, there is no asymptotic efficiency gain to analyze the original data when the parameter of main interest has a common value across studies and the summary statistics are based on maximum likelihood theory regardless of different nuisance parameters among studies when the nuisance parameters have distinct values. The authors also demonstrated their results with simulations from the logistic regression setting. The R code for this simulation can be found from `http://www.bios.unc.edu/~dzeng/Meta.html`. Note that this conclusion generally fails to hold when the nuisance parameters have common values as discussed in Lin and Zeng (2010) and Simmonds and Higgins (2007).

In the next section, we follow this paper to design a simulation study following the continuous data structure reported from the Lamotrigine clinical studies.

8.5 Simulation Study on Continuous Outcomes

We do not reproduce the theoretical work from Lin and Zeng (2010) because it is available from the literature for interested readers. This paper demonstrated theoretically and numerically that there is little or no efficiency gain of IPD over meta-analysis - gives assurance to performing a meta-analysis using summary statistics. The practical implications from this work regarding whether to use IPD or meta-analysis are noted and emphasized. Usually patient level data are not available for analysis and may be difficult and costly to obtain if available. In this section, we further illustrate this conclusion from a simulation based on the Lamotrigine clinical studies.

8.5.1 Simulation Data Generator

We simulate data from K studies. Each of these studies includes two treatments, which are named treatment (`TRT`) and placebo (`PBO`), with n_i study participants from each study randomly assigned to these 2 treatments with binomial probability distribution of $p = 0.5$. The $nvec$ denotes the vector of sample size from these K studies, i.e. $nvec = (n_1, \cdots, n_K)$. Similarly, we denote $meanvec$ and $sdvec$ as the vectors of means and standard deviations from these K studies.

For simplicity, we simulate data from a fixed-effects model setting where the model is

$$y_{ij} = \mu + \epsilon_{ij} \tag{8.1}$$

where i indexes the ith study ($i = 1, \cdots, K$) and j for observations within study ($j = 1, \cdots, n_i$), and μ is the same for all K studies in the fixed-effects model, but different for each treatment. This setting can be easily modified for a random-effects model by adding an extra term μ_i to μ to simulate variation and heterogeneity among studies and we leave this to interested readers.

In this case, we can build a data simulator (called `data.generator`) to generate data from K studies with two treatments as follows:

```
> # The function for data generation
> data.generator =  function(K, nvec, meanvec, sdvec){
 # Initialize data generation
 trt = study = mu = epsilon = NULL;
 # Loop to generate data for each study
 for(i in 1:K){
        # study identifier
        study = append(study,rep(i, nvec[i]))
        # indicator for treatment assignment
        trt0 = mu0 = which.trt = rbinom(nvec[i],1,0.5)
        # assign 1 to TRT and get its mean value
        trt0[mu0==1] = 1; mu0[mu0==1] = meanvec[i]
        # assign 0 for Placebo and get its mean value
        trt0[mu0==0] = 0; mu0[mu0==0] = meanvec[i+K]
        # epsilion
        epsilon0 = rnorm(nvec[i], 0, sdvec)
        # put together
        trt  = append(trt,trt0)
        mu   = append(mu, mu0)
        epsilon = append(epsilon, epsilon0)
                } # end of i-loop for data generation
 # Put the data into a dataframe
 trt[trt==1] = "TRT"
 trt[trt==0] = "PBO"
 y   = mu + epsilon
 dat = data.frame(Study=as.factor(study), TRT = trt,mu=mu,y=y)
 # Output the dataframe
 dat
 } # end of function "data.generator"
```

As an example, let's follow the Lamotrigine clinical studies to generate data with inputs as follows:

```
> # Set the seed for reproducibility
> set.seed(123)
> # The number of studies
> K    = 4
> # The number of observations for each study
> n    = 200
> nvec = rep(n, K)
> # Print it to show the sample size
> nvec

[1] 200 200 200 200

> # Treatment means from HAMD in Lamotrigine clinical study
> mTRT    = -10; mPBO = -8
> meanvec = c(rep(mTRT,K), rep(mPBO,K))
> # SDs for each study
> sdvec   = 8 + runif(K)
> sdvec

[1] 8.29 8.79 8.41 8.88
```

The SD for HAMD is close to 8 in the real data and we add values from a random uniform distribution to simulate study-level heterogeneity in this simulation. With these inputs, we call `data.generator` to generate individual patient level data as follows:

```
> # Call `data.generator'
> dat =  data.generator(K,nvec,meanvec,sdvec)
> # Print the first few rows of data
> head(dat)

  Study TRT  mu     y
1     1 TRT -10 -12.0
2     1 PBO  -8 -11.1
3     1 TRT -10 -18.0
```

```
4       1 TRT -10 -10.4
5       1 TRT -10 -16.5
6       1 PBO  -8 -22.7
```

This dataframe "dat" would have $4 \times 200 = 800$ observations with 4 columns as Study to denote the $K = 4$ studies, TRT to denote the treatment assignments, mu as the simulated true means and y is the individual-level data from equation 8.1. We use R function head to see the *head* six data lines. The distribution of the generated data can be graphically illustrated in Figure 8.3 using R function bwplot as follows:

```
> print(bwplot(y~Study|TRT, data=dat,xlab="Study", lwd=3,
 ylab="Simulated Data",cex=1.3,pch=20,type=c("p", "r")))
```

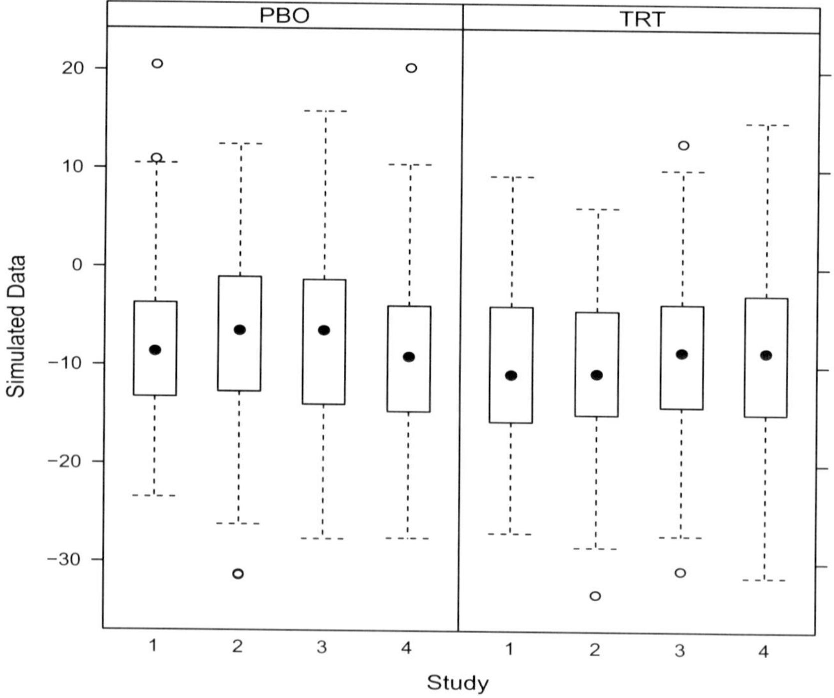

FIGURE 8.3: Simulated Data from Four Studies

8.5.2 Simulation Data Estimator

With the data generated from Section 8.5.1, we then estimate the relevant parameters from both IPD and MA models and design an estimator which is named as `data.estimator`. For this estimator, we design and contrast three analysis models. The first model is the analysis of variance model for each study which is in fact the t-test in this simulation since there are only two treatments. This analysis is to be compared with the study-wise z-test in meta-analysis. The second model is an analysis model to pool the data from the K studies with model formulation of $y = \mu + TRT + Study + \epsilon$. The third model is the fixed-effects meta-analysis model which is used to compare results with the analysis model with pooled data. For the purpose of this simulation and estimation, we mainly keep track of the estimation results from treatment effect on the parameter estimates, standard errors and the associated p-values from both IPD and MA models.

The input for this `data.estimator` would be the `dat` from `data.simulator` from Section 8.5.1. The R implementation is as follows:

```
> # The function of `estimator'
> data.estimator = function(dat){
 # 1. Get the study ID from the dataframe
 idStudy = unique(dat$Study)
 nStudy  = length(idStudy)
 # 2. loop to get p-values for each study
 eachIPD.pval = rep(0, nStudy)
 for(i in 1:nStudy){
 m4Study = lm(y~TRT, data=dat[dat$Study==idStudy[i],])
 eachIPD.pval[i] = summary(m4Study)$coef[2,4]
                  } # end of i-loop
 # 3. The IPD with pooled data using linear model
 mIPD         = lm(y~TRT+Study,dat)
 # Extract parms from IPD model
 poolIPD.trt.p   = anova(mIPD)["TRT","Pr(>F)"]
 poolIPD.study.p = anova(mIPD)["Study","Pr(>F)"]
 poolIPD.trt.est = summary(mIPD)$coef["TRTTRT","Estimate"]
 poolIPD.trt.se  = summary(mIPD)$coef["TRTTRT","Std. Error"]
```

```
# 4. Meta-analysis
# 4.1. Aggregate the individual level data into study-level
ndat =aggregate(dat$y,list(Study=dat$Study,TRT=dat$TRT),length)
mdat =aggregate(dat$y,list(Study=dat$Study,TRT=dat$TRT),mean)
sddat=aggregate(dat$y,list(Study=dat$Study,TRT=dat$TRT),sd)
# 4.2. Call the library
library(metafor)
# 4.3 Calculate the ESs
esdat = escalc(measure="MD",
        n1i = ndat$x[ndat$TRT=="TRT"],
        n2i = ndat$x[ndat$TRT=="PBO"],
        m1i = mdat$x[mdat$TRT=="TRT"],
        m2i = mdat$x[mdat$TRT=="PBO"],
        sd1i= sddat$x[sddat$TRT=="TRT"],
        sd2i= sddat$x[sddat$TRT=="PBO"], append=T)
rownames(esdat) = ndat$Study[ndat$TRT=="TRT"]
# 4.4. z- and p-values for IPD in each study
z               = esdat$yi/sqrt(esdat$vi)
pval.studywise = 2*(1-pnorm(abs(z)))
# 4.5. Fixed-effects meta-analysis
meta.MD.FE = rma(yi,vi,measure="MD",method="FE", data=esdat)
# 4.6. Extract the estimate, p-values for ES and heterogeneity
MA.muhat.FE   = meta.MD.FE$b
MA.muhatse.FE = meta.MD.FE$se
MA.p.FE       = meta.MD.FE$pval
MA.pQ.FE      = meta.MD.FE$QEp
# 5. output from the estimator
out = list(
eachIPD.pval   = eachIPD.pval,
pval.studywise = pval.studywise,
IPD.trt.est    = poolIPD.trt.est,
IPD.trt.se     = poolIPD.trt.se,
IPD.trt.p      = poolIPD.trt.p,
IPD.study.p    = poolIPD.study.p,
MA.muhat.FE    = MA.muhat.FE,
```

```
MA.muhatse.FE  = MA.muhatse.FE,
MA.p.FE        = MA.p.FE,
MA.pQ.FE       = MA.pQ.FE)
# 6. Return the output
out
} # end of "data.estimator"
```

With this estimator, we call the function for the data we generated in Section 8.5.1 as follows:

```
> data.estimator(dat)

$eachIPD.pval
[1] 0.18036 0.00179 0.15436 0.98132


$pval.studywise
[1] 0.17821 0.00151 0.15149 0.98131
attr(,"measure")
[1] "MD"


$IPD.trt.est
[1] -1.76


$IPD.trt.se
[1] 0.604


$IPD.trt.p
[1] 0.00348


$IPD.study.p
[1] 0.764


$MA.muhat.FE
         [,1]
intrcpt -1.81


$MA.muhatse.FE
```

```
[1] 0.601

$MA.p.FE
[1] 0.00259

$MA.pQ.FE
[1] 0.183
```

As can be seen from the output for individual-studywise, only the second study is statistically significant and the other three are not. But when the four studies are pooled in IPD model, the estimated treatment difference is `IPD.trt.est` = -1.76 with standard error of `IPD.trt.se` = 0.604 and the associated p-value of `IPD.trt.p` = 0.00348. In addition, the associated p-value for study-effect is `IPD.study.p` = 0.764. Comparatively from the meta-analysis, the estimated treatment difference is `MA.muhat.FE` = -1.81 with standard error of `MA.muhatse.FE` = 0.601 and associated p-value of `MA.p.FE` = 0.00259. The associated p-value for study heterogeneity is `MA.pQ.FE`=0.183.

8.5.3 Simulation

With the data generator in Section 8.5.1 and estimator in Section 8.5.2, we now run a large number of simulations to compare treatment effects as well as efficiency for both the IPD and MA models.

In order to effectively run the simulation, we develop another R function which is named `IPD2MA`, run the extensive simulations and save the results for further graphical illustration and model comparison. This function has inputs from the `data.generator` with an additional input for the number of simulations which is denoted by `nsim`. This function is as follows with detailed annotations:

```
> # Main function for the simulation
> IPD2MA = function(nsim,K,nvec,meanvec,sdvec)
 {
 # Put program checkers
 if(length(nvec)!= K)
   cat("Wrong for the number of obs in each study","\n")
```

```
if(length(meanvec)!= 2*K)
  cat("Wrong for the study mean setup","\n")
if(length(sdvec)!= K)
  cat("Wrong for the study SD setup","\n")

# Output initialization
IPD.trt.est=IPD.trt.se= IPD.trt.p=IPD.study.p =
MA.muhat.FE=MA.muhatse.FE=MA.p.FE=MA.pQ.FE=rep(0, nsim)
# Now loop-over for "nsim" simulation and extract the measures
for(s in 1:nsim){
cat("Simulating iteration =",s,sep=" ", "\n\n")
        # call "data.generator" to generate data
        dat = data.generator(K, nvec, meanvec, sdvec)
        # call estimator to get estimates from IPD and MA
        est = data.estimator(dat)
        # Extract the measures from the IPD and MA analyses
        IPD.trt.est[s]  = est$IPD.trt.est
    IPD.trt.se[s]   = est$IPD.trt.se
        IPD.trt.p[s]    = est$IPD.trt.p
    IPD.study.p[s]  = est$IPD.study.p
        MA.muhat.FE[s]  = est$MA.muhat.FE
    MA.muhatse.FE[s]= est$MA.muhatse.FE
    MA.p.FE[s]      = est$MA.p.FE
    MA.pQ.FE[s]     = est$MA.pQ.FE
        } #end of s-loop
# Summary statistics
out = data.frame(
IPD.trt.est   = IPD.trt.est,    IPD.trt.se    = IPD.trt.se,
IPD.trt.p     = IPD.trt.p,      IPD.study.p   = IPD.study.p,
MA.muhat.FE   = MA.muhat.FE,    MA.muhatse.FE = MA.muhatse.FE,
MA.p.FE       = MA.p.FE,        MA.pQ.FE      = MA.pQ.FE)
# Return the dataframe "out"
out
} # end of "IPD2meta"
```

With the same inputs from Section 8.5.1, we run a simulation with 100,000 replications (note that if your computer is slower, you can reduce the number of simulations to 10,000) as follows:

```
> # The number of simulations
> nsim =100000
> # Call "IPD2MA" to run simulations
> IPD2MA.simu = IPD2MA(nsim,K,nvec,meanvec,sdvec)
```

This produces a dataframe named `IPD2MA.simu` to hold the 100,000 simulation results which includes 8 columns from both IPD and MA models. We now compare the performance between IPD and MA models with this dataframe. We first investigate the efficiency as noted in Lin and Zeng (2010) along with the estimates for treatment effect. The efficiency is defined as the ratio of estimated variance for the treatment effect between IPD and MA models - which is the squared value of the estimated standard errors and denoted by `relEff`. We also consider the relative estimates of treatment effect which is defined as the ratio of the estimates between IPD and MA models and denoted by `relEst`. We output the mean and mode along with the 95% CI from these 100,000 simulations using the following R code chunk:

```
> # The relative efficiency
> relEff = IPD2MA.simu$IPD.trt.se^2/IPD2MA.simu$MA.muhatse.FE^2
> # The mean
> mean(relEff)

[1] 1.01

> # The mode and 95% CI
> quantile(relEff, c(0.025, 0.5,0.975))

 2.5%   50% 97.5%
 0.99  1.01  1.03

> # The relative estimate
> relEst= IPD2MA.simu$IPD.trt.est/IPD2MA.simu$MA.muhat.FE
> # The mean
> mean(relEst)
```

```
[1] 1
```

```
> # The mode and 95% CI
> quantile(relEst, c(0.025, 0.5,0.975))
```

```
 2.5%   50% 97.5%
0.936 1.000 1.072
```

It can be seen that the mean and mode for the relative efficiency are both 1.01 with 95% CI of (0.99, 1.03) which indicates that both IPD and MA models have comparable efficiency and are consistent with the finding from Lin and Zeng (2010). Further, the mean and mode for the relative estimates for treatment effect are both 1 with 95% CI of (0.936, 1.072) which again indicates the comparability between IPD and MA models. The distributions for both the relative efficiency and relative estimates for treatment effect can be graphically illustrated using `boxplot` as seen in Figure 8.4 which can be produced using following R code chunk:

```
> # Call boxplot to plot the relative efficiency and estimates
> par(mfrow=c(1,2))
> boxplot(relEff, main="Relative Efficiency",
        las=1,ylim=c(0.98,1.04))
> boxplot(relEst, main="Relative Treatment Estimates",
        las=1,ylim=c(0.93,1.07))
```

Apart from the above comparable relative measures, we also compare the number of simulations among these 100,000 simulations that report a statistically significant treatment effect which can be calculated as follows:

```
> # For IPD
> n4TRT.IPD = sum(IPD2MA.simu$IPD.trt.p<0.05)
> n4TRT.IPD
```

```
[1] 90606
```

```
> # For MA
> n4TRT.MA  = sum(IPD2MA.simu$MA.p.FE<0.05)
> n4TRT.MA
```

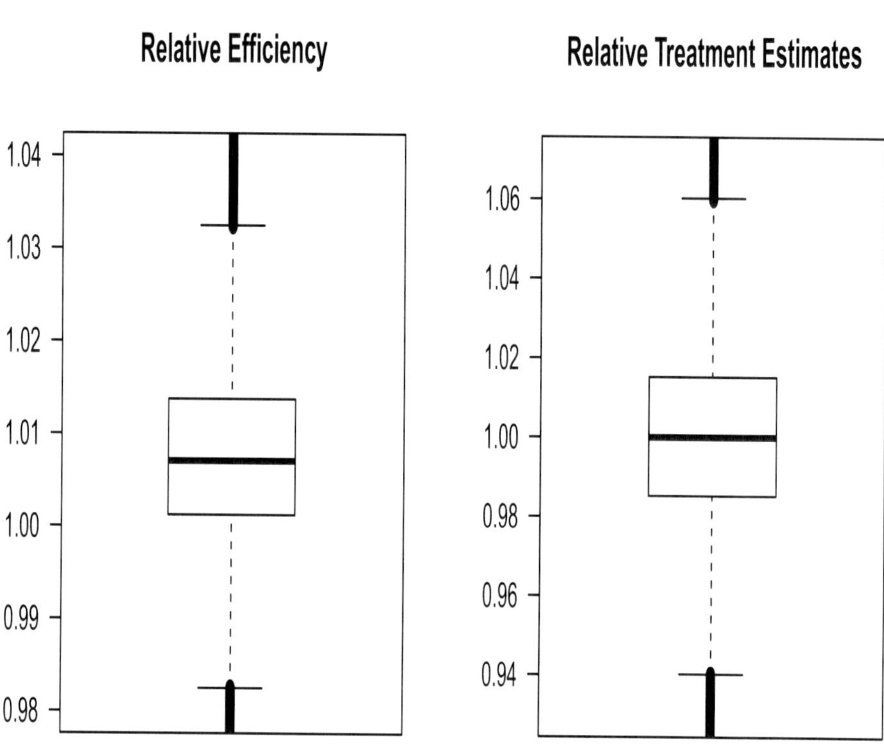

FIGURE 8.4: Distributions for the Relative Efficiency and Relative Estimates

```
[1] 90643
```

It can be seen that the number of simulations among these 100,000 simulations that report significant treatment effect is 90,606 from the IPD pooled model and 90,643 from the meta-analysis. Therefore both models give similar results for testing treatment effect. The same can be done for testing heterogeneity among studies with following R code chunk:

```
> # for IPD
> n4Study.IPD = sum(IPD2MA.simu$IPD.study.p<0.05)
> n4Study.IPD
```

```
[1] 5027
```

```
> # For MA
> n4Study.MA   = sum(IPD2MA.simu$MA.pQ.FE<0.05)
> n4Study.MA
```

```
[1] 5158
```

Again, very compatible results are obtained for both models.

8.6 Discussion

In this chapter, we started with real individual patient-level data on lamotrigine to treat bipolar depression in comparison to a placebo to illustrate the pros and cons of IPD and MA. A series of models were used to analyze this data and we concluded that both models yielded similar conclusions that lamotrigine is more effective than placebo in treating bipolar depression.

This analysis served as another real example for the conclusions reported in Lin and Zeng (2010). We further designed a simulation study using the data structure from the lamotrigine clinical studies and simulated 100,000 replications to compare the relative efficiency and the relative parameter estimates on treatment effects as well as the number of simulations that yielded statistically significant treatment effects. All demonstrated that both models yielded very comparable results.

This chapter thus serves to further promote meta-analysis using study-level summary statistics. Without much loss in relative efficiency for testing treatment effect, MA is recommended since it is usually difficult to obtain original individual-level data and is costlier and more time-consuming.

Comparing the performance of IPD and MA models has received considerable debate in the meta-analysis literature. Olkin and Sampson (1998) and Mathew and Nordstrom (1999) showed their equivalence in comparing multiple treatments and a control. The theoretical results in Lin and Zeng (2010) are more general in this area as discussed in the paper.

A novel *confidence distributions* approach was proposed in Singh et al. (2005), Xie et al. (2011) and Xie and Singh (2013) to unify the framework for meta-analysis. This approach uses a (data-dependent) distribution function, instead of the point (point estimator) or interval (confidence interval), to estimate the parameter of interest which then led to new development in meta-analysis. An associated R package `gmeta` is created by Guang Yang, Pixu Shi and Minge Xie which is available at `http://stat.rutgers.edu/home/gyang/researches/gmetaRpackage/`. In his Ph.D. dissertation (`http://mss3.libraries.rutgers.edu/dlr/showfed.php?pid=rutgers-lib:37435`), Dr. Dungang Liu utilized this *confidence distributions* and developed an effective and efficient approach to combine heterogeneous studies. He showed that the new method can combine studies different in populations, designs or outcomes, including the cases pointed out in Sutton and Higgins (2008) and Whitehead et al. (1999). He showed theoretically and numerically that his approach was asymptotically as efficient as the maximum likelihood approach using individual-level data from all the studies. However different from the IPD analysis, his approach only requires summary statistics from relevant studies and does not require the individual-level data. Several examples and cases were considered in this dissertation along with his theoretical theorems. We recommend this method to interested readers.

Other reviews on this topic can be found in Simmonds et al. (2005) and Lyman and Kuderer (2005).

Chapter 9

Meta-Analysis for Rare Events

All the methods presented thus far for meta-analysis in this book are based on large sample theory as well as the theory of large sample approximations. For rare events, these methods usually break down. For example, when events are zeros, the methods for risk-ratio and odds-ratio discussed in Section 4.2 cannot be used and when the events are rare, but not all zeros, the variance estimates for these methods are not robust which may lead to unreliable statistical inferences. The typical remedies are to remove the studies with zero events from the meta analysis, or add a small value, say 0.5, to the rare events which could lead to biased statistical inferences as pointed out by Tian et al. (2009) and Cai et al. (2010).

In this chapter, we use the well-known Rosiglitazone meta-analysis data to illustrate the bias when classical meta-analysis methods are used for rare events. We then introduce a R package `gmeta` which implements a novel `confidence distributions` approach proposed in Singh et al. (2005), Xie et al. (2011) and Xie and Singh (2013) to unify the framework for meta-analysis where two methods are implemented for meta-analysis of rare events. The general introduction to this package can be found from `http://stat.rutgers.edu/home/gyang/researches/gmetaRpackage/`. As seen from this link, methods implemented in `gmeta` include:

1. Combination of p-values: Fisher's method, Stouffer (normal) method, Tippett (min) method, Max method, Sum method;

2. Model based meta-analysis methods: Fixed-effect model, Random-effect model, Robust method1 (a small number of large studies), Robust method2 (a large number of small studies);

3. Combine evidence from 2 by 2 tables: Mantel-Haenszel Odds Ratio,

Peto's Log Odds Ratio, Exact method1 (Odd Ratio), Exact method2 (Risk Difference)

Among these methods, the 'Exact method1' (i.e. `exact1`) for odds-ratio as detailed in `http://mss3.libraries.rutgers.edu/dlr/showfed.php?pid=rutgers-lib:37435` and the 'Exact method2' (i.e. `exact2`) in Tian et al. (2009) for risk-difference can be used for rare event meta-analysis.

9.1 The Rosiglitazone Meta-Analysis

In a meta-analysis for the effect of rosiglitazone on the risk of myocardial infarction (MI) and death from cardiovascular causes, Nissen and Wolski (2007) searched the available published literature and found 116 potentially relevant studies where 42 of these met the inclusion criteria. Data were then extracted from the 42 publications and combined using a fixed-effects meta-analysis model. This yielded an odds-ratio for the rosiglitazone group to the control group of 1.43 with 95% CI of (1.03, 1.98) and p-value $= 0.03$ for MI; and 1.64 with 95% CI of (0.98, 2.74) and p-value $= 0.06$ for death from cardiovascular causes. Based on these results, the authors concluded that rosiglitazone use was statistically significantly associated with risk of myocardial infarction, and was borderline statistically significant with death from cardiovascular causes. Therefore using rosiglitazone for the treatment of Type-2 diabetes could lead to serious adverse cardiovascular effects.

Since its publication, numerous authors questioned the validity of the analysis and interpretation of the results. For example, Shuster and Schatz (2008) (which is online available at `http://care.diabetesjournals.org/content/31/3/e10.full.pdf`) pointed out that the fixed-effects meta-analysis was inappropriate. They reanalyzed 48 (not 42) eligible studies via a new random-effects method (Shuster et al., 2007) that yielded different conclusions; i.e. a strong association with cardiac death was found, but there was no significant association with myocardial infarction. Other meta-analyses of data from the studies can be found from Dahabreh (2008), Tian et al. (2009),

Cai et al. (2010) and Lane (2012) (online publication available at http://www.ncbi.nlm.nih.gov/pubmed/22218366).

In this chapter, we further illustrate meta-analysis for rare events using this data with R implementations in gmeta.

9.2 Step-by-Step Data Analysis in R

9.2.1 Load the Data

The data from Tian et al. (2009), which is available as the supplementary material at http://www.ncbi.nlm.nih.gov/pmc/articles/PMC2648899/bin/kxn034_index.html, are re-entered into our Excel databook (i.e. dat4Meta). This data can be loaded into R with the following R code chunk:

```
> # Load the Rosiglitazone data from excel file
> require(gdata)
> # Get the data path
> datfile = "Your Data Path/dat4Meta.xls"
> # Call "read.xls" to read the Excel data
> dat  = read.xls(datfile, sheet="Data.Rosiglitazone",
                  perl="c:/perl64/bin/perl.exe")
> # Print the first 6 studies
> head(dat)
```

```
ID  Study  n.TRT MI.TRT Death.TRT n.CTRL MI.CTRL Death.CTRL
1 49653/011  357    2        1      176       0     0
2 49653/020  391    2        0      207       1     0
3 49653/024  774    1        0      185       1     0
4 49653/093  213    0        0      109       1     0
5 49653/094  232    1        1      116       0     0
6     100684  43    0        0       47       1     0
```

With this dataframe, we perform meta-analyses of both the risk difference (RD) and odds-ratio (OR) for myocardial infarction (MI) and cardiovascular death (Death). We contrast the results from the classical fixed-effects and random-effects models using the R package `meta` to the results from the *confidence distribution* (CD) implemented in the R package `gmeta`.

9.2.2 Data Analysis for Myocardial Infarction (MI)

To analyze the data for MI, we first create a dataframe (only for MI) as follows:

```
> datMI     = dat[,c("MI.TRT","MI.CTRL","n.TRT","n.CTRL")]
```

For classical fixed-effects and random-effects meta-analysis, we make use of the R library `meta`, introduced in previous chapters, and use the inverse weighting method to combine studies. This is implemented in the following R code chunk:

```
> # Load the library
> library(meta)
> # Call metabin with RD=risk difference
> MI.RD.wo = metabin(MI.TRT,n.TRT,MI.CTRL,n.CTRL,data=datMI,
        incr=0, method="Inverse", sm="RD")
> # Print the summary
> summary(MI.RD.wo)

Number of studies combined: k=48

                           RD           95%-CI    z  p.value
Fixed effect model    0.002  [0.001; 0.003] 3.24   0.0012
Random effects model 0.002  [0.001; 0.003] 3.24   0.0012

Quantifying heterogeneity:
tau^2 < 0.0001; H = 1 [1; 1]; I^2 = 0% [0%; 0%]

Test of heterogeneity:
    Q d.f.  p.value
```

```
27.9   47   0.9879

Details on meta-analytical method:
- Inverse variance method
- DerSimonian-Laird estimator for tau^2
```

As seen from the summary, the combined RD = 0.0018 with 95% CI of (7e-04, 0.0028) and a p-value = 0.0012 for both fixed-effects and random-effects models - since the `Test of heterogeneity` is not statistically significant (p-value = 0.9879 and $\hat{\tau}^2 \approx 0$). Even though the RD is small and the left endpoint of the CI is just to the right of 0, these results are consistent with the conclusion that MIs in rosiglitazone group are statistically significantly higher than in the control group.

Note that in the above R code chunk, the option `incr` is set to zero which means no value is added to the zero MIs. In this dataframe, there are 10 studies with zero MIs for both rosiglitazone and control. The standard errors for the RD corresponding to these studies cannot be computed which is set to zero as default in this R function call.

A typical way to adjust the zero MIs is to add a small increment of 0.5 to them as a correction for lack of continuity, which is the default setting in the R function call to `metabin` as follows:

```
> # Call metabin with default setting to add 0.5
> MI.RD = metabin(MI.TRT,n.TRT,MI.CTRL,n.CTRL,data=datMI,
          method="Inverse", sm="RD")
> # Print the summary
> summary(MI.RD)

Number of studies combined: k=48

                         RD       95%-CI     z  p.value
Fixed effect model    0.001  [0; 0.003] 1.73   0.0834
Random effects model 0.001  [0; 0.003] 1.73   0.0834

Quantifying heterogeneity:
tau^2 < 0.0001; H = 1 [1; 1]; I^2 = 0% [0%; 0%]
```

```
Test of heterogeneity:
     Q d.f. p.value
 17.98   47       1

Details on meta-analytical method:
- Inverse variance method
- DerSimonian-Laird estimator for tau^2
```

With 0.5 added to the zero cells, we see from the output that the combined RD is now 0.0014 with 95% CI of (-2e-04, 0.0029) and p-value $= 0.0834$ for both fixed-effects and random-effects models. The conclusion changed from statistically significant to statistically non-significant. Readers may want to try to add different increments to the zero cells and examine the effects of this artificial correction (although well founded in history of the analysis of contingency table data) for lack of continuity. In fact, Sweeting et al. (2004) provided compelling evidence that imputing arbitrary numbers to zero cells in continuity correction can result in very different conclusions.

Tian et al. (2009) developed an exact and efficient inference procedure to use all the data without this artificial continuity correction. This is a special case of the *confidence distribution* (CD) framework as proved in the **Supplementary Notes** at `http://stat.rutgers.edu/home/gyang/researches/gmetaRpackage/`. This method is implemented into `gmeta` as `method="exact2"`. The R code to implement this method is as follows:

```
> # Call "gmeta" with method="exact2"
> MI.exactTianRD =  gmeta(datMI,gmi.type="2x2",method="exact2",
          ci.level=0.95,n=2000)
```

The summary of this modeling can be printed as follows:

```
> summary(MI.exactTianRD)

       Exact Meta-Analysis Approach through CD-Framework
Call:
gmeta.default(gmi = datMI, gmi.type = "2x2", method = "exact2",
```

```
    n = 2000, ci.level = 0.95)

Combined CD Summary:
               mean    median  stddev     CI.1     CI.2
exp1      -4.53e-03 -5.81e-03 0.00619 -0.01777 0.020567
exp2       6.12e-04 -1.16e-03 0.00878 -0.01396 0.018077
exp3       5.97e-03  3.73e-03 0.00727 -0.00565 0.025406
exp4       1.12e-02  1.05e-02 0.01256 -0.01489 0.044330
exp5      -2.44e-03 -4.30e-03 0.00819 -0.01949 0.031133
exp6       1.75e-02  1.95e-02 0.03239       NA       NA
exp7      -7.89e-03 -7.47e-03 0.01245 -0.03842 0.029153
exp8      -2.24e-02 -3.27e-02 0.02650       NA 0.027238
exp9      -2.50e-03 -2.56e-03 0.00389 -0.01194 0.009509
exp10     -1.84e-03 -4.05e-03 0.00694 -0.01605 0.026811
exp11      3.49e-03  3.79e-03 0.00504 -0.01164 0.016145
exp12     -1.53e-03 -3.44e-03 0.00622 -0.01209 0.017555
exp13     -3.08e-03 -5.39e-03 0.01073 -0.02021 0.012985
exp14     -3.91e-03 -4.61e-03 0.00536 -0.01519 0.017104
exp15      1.00e-03 -1.08e-03 0.00861 -0.01378 0.019149
exp16      5.87e-03  5.62e-03 0.01363 -0.01808 0.039631
exp17      9.03e-03  6.97e-03 0.02226 -0.03358 0.055565
exp18     -7.81e-03 -9.18e-03 0.01055 -0.02966 0.033602
exp19     -1.35e-02 -1.61e-02 0.01769 -0.05159 0.025194
exp20      2.48e-03 -3.53e-04 0.00951 -0.01477 0.030524
exp21      8.63e-03  7.78e-03 0.01272 -0.02793 0.040218
exp22      6.09e-03  5.53e-03 0.00878 -0.01952 0.028042
exp23     -1.46e-02 -1.71e-02 0.02632       NA       NA
exp24     -1.49e-02 -2.85e-02 0.03846       NA 0.049259
exp25      8.28e-03  7.01e-03 0.00615 -0.00254 0.023689
exp26      7.00e-03  5.72e-03 0.02451 -0.04541       NA
exp27     -6.34e-03 -7.63e-03 0.01003 -0.03105 0.025329
exp28     -4.22e-03 -4.17e-03 0.00649 -0.01995 0.015046
exp29     -1.03e-02 -1.18e-02 0.01668 -0.05235 0.040833
exp30     -5.72e-03 -5.40e-03 0.00893 -0.02750 0.021104
exp31      2.79e-03 -1.43e-06 0.01502 -0.02461 0.047615
```

```
exp32        -9.28e-05 -8.58e-04 0.00241 -0.00421 0.009685
exp33         8.12e-04 -8.25e-05 0.00287 -0.00417 0.009115
exp34         5.67e-03  3.73e-03 0.01191 -0.01673 0.030232
exp35        -3.27e-03 -3.84e-03 0.00512 -0.01577 0.013017
exp36        -3.90e-03 -4.15e-03 0.00592 -0.01818 0.013397
exp37        -1.72e-03 -3.43e-03 0.00589 -0.01445 0.023542
exp38         1.56e-04 -1.94e-04 0.00651 -0.01712 0.018428
exp39         6.13e-04 -2.07e-03 0.00806 -0.01238 0.024941
exp40        -2.41e-04 -2.33e-03 0.00715 -0.01234 0.021490
exp41        -2.39e-03 -2.52e-03 0.00200 -0.00651 0.001540
exp42        -4.70e-03 -4.70e-03 0.00445 -0.01419 0.003493
exp43         2.94e-03 -6.03e-07 0.01802 -0.02813 0.056682
exp44         2.10e-03 -1.27e-04 0.00812 -0.01255 0.025546
exp45        -3.43e-04 -5.37e-04 0.01453 -0.03956 0.038902
exp46        -8.29e-05 -4.24e-03 0.04255       NA       NA
exp47         1.16e-04 -5.10e-07 0.00532 -0.01408 0.015145
exp48         1.43e-03 -1.07e-05 0.00424 -0.00507 0.013882
combined.cd -1.77e-03 -2.21e-03 0.00188 -0.00386 0.000878

Confidence level= 0.95
```

The last row contains the combined estimates and can be produced as follows:

```
> summary(MI.exactTianRD)$mms[49,]

                 mean    median  stddev     CI.1     CI.2
combined.cd -0.00177 -0.00221 0.00188 -0.00386 0.000878
```

We see that the mean difference is -0.00177 with 95% CI of (-0.00386, 0.00088) indicating no statistically significantly difference between rosiglitazone group and the control group on MI.

We now analyze the MI dataframe using the odds ratio. Similarly, the classical fixed-effects and random-effects models can be implemented as follows:

```
> # Call metabin without 0.5 correction
```

```
> MI.OR.wo = metabin(MI.TRT,n.TRT,MI.CTRL,n.CTRL,data=datMI,
        incr=0,method="Inverse", sm="OR")
> # Summary
> summary(MI.OR.wo)

Number of studies combined: k=38

                        OR           95%-CI    z  p.value
Fixed effect model    1.29  [0.895; 1.85] 1.36   0.1736
Random effects model 1.29  [0.895; 1.85] 1.36   0.1736

Quantifying heterogeneity:
tau^2 < 0.0001; H = 1 [1; 1]; I^2 = 0% [0%; 0%]

Test of heterogeneity:
   Q d.f. p.value
 5.7   37       1

Details on meta-analytical method:
- Inverse variance method
- DerSimonian-Laird estimator for tau^2


> # Call metabin with default 0.5 correction
> MI.OR = metabin(MI.TRT,n.TRT,MI.CTRL,n.CTRL,data=datMI,
            method="Inverse", sm="OR")
> # Print the Summary
> summary(MI.OR)

Number of studies combined: k=38

                        OR          95%-CI    z  p.value
Fixed effect model    1.29  [0.94; 1.76] 1.57   0.1161
Random effects model 1.29  [0.94; 1.76] 1.57   0.1161

Quantifying heterogeneity:
```

```
tau^2 < 0.0001; H = 1 [1; 1]; I^2 = 0% [0%; 0%]

Test of heterogeneity:
     Q d.f.  p.value
 16.22   37   0.9988

Details on meta-analytical method:
- Inverse variance method
- DerSimonian-Laird estimator for tau^2
```

We see that with or without the default 0.5 continuity correction, the 95% CIs and p-values are slightly different, but yield the same conclusion that there is no statistically significantly difference between the rosiglitazone group and the control group on MI.

We now can call gmeta for the exact method using the odds ratio, which is implemented as follows:

```
> # Call "gmeta" for "exact1" on OR
> MI.exactLiuOR = gmeta(datMI,gmi.type="2x2",
         method="exact1", ci.level=0.95,n=2000)
> # Print the summary
> summary(MI.exactLiuOR)

       Exact Meta-Analysis Approach through CD-Framework
Call:
gmeta.default(gmi = datMI, gmi.type = "2x2", method = "exact1",
    n = 2000, ci.level = 0.95)

Combined CD Summary:
                 mean  median stddev   CI.1  CI.2
exp1              Inf      NA    Inf -1.951   Inf
exp2           0.1141 -0.0044  1.360 -2.525 3.446
exp3          -1.4316 -1.4333  1.631 -5.110 2.233
exp4             -Inf      NA    Inf   -Inf 2.274
exp5              Inf      NA    Inf -3.636   Inf
exp6             -Inf      NA    Inf   -Inf 3.033
```

```
exp7        Inf      NA   Inf -2.920   Inf
exp8     0.9942  0.9346 0.888 -0.669 3.002
exp9        Inf      NA   Inf -2.939   Inf
exp10       Inf      NA   Inf -3.687   Inf
exp11      -Inf      NA   Inf   -Inf 2.971
exp12       Inf      NA   Inf -2.625   Inf
exp13    0.7556  0.6374 1.360 -1.882 4.088
exp14       Inf      NA   Inf -1.922   Inf
exp15    0.0593 -0.0592 1.360 -2.581 3.392
exp16   -0.6514 -0.6520 1.634 -4.320 3.018
exp17   -0.8065 -0.6886 1.366 -4.143 1.840
exp18       Inf      NA   Inf -1.928   Inf
exp19    1.1847  1.0326 1.266 -1.135 4.398
exp20       NaN      NA   Inf   -Inf   Inf
exp21      -Inf      NA   Inf   -Inf 2.928
exp22      -Inf      NA   Inf   -Inf 2.933
exp23       Inf      NA   Inf -2.909   Inf
exp24       Inf      NA   Inf -2.970   Inf
exp25      -Inf      NA   Inf   -Inf 0.534
exp26   -0.4690 -0.4347 0.978 -2.603 1.466
exp27       Inf      NA   Inf -2.979   Inf
exp28       Inf      NA   Inf -2.898   Inf
exp29       Inf      NA   Inf -2.956   Inf
exp30       Inf      NA   Inf -2.921   Inf
exp31       NaN      NA   Inf   -Inf   Inf
exp32       Inf      NA   Inf -4.084   Inf
exp33       NaN      NA   Inf   -Inf   Inf
exp34   -0.8514 -0.7333 1.362 -4.183 1.788
exp35       Inf      NA   Inf -2.973   Inf
exp36       Inf      NA   Inf -2.876   Inf
exp37       Inf      NA   Inf -3.656   Inf
exp38       NaN      NA   Inf   -Inf   Inf
exp39       Inf      NA   Inf -4.306   Inf
exp40       Inf      NA   Inf -4.107   Inf
exp41    0.5133  0.5055 0.428 -0.314 1.385
```

```
exp42         0.2739  0.2760  0.251 -0.226 0.762
exp43            NaN      NA    Inf   -Inf   Inf
exp44            NaN      NA    Inf   -Inf   Inf
exp45            NaN      NA    Inf   -Inf   Inf
exp46            NaN      NA    Inf   -Inf   Inf
exp47            NaN      NA    Inf   -Inf   Inf
exp48            NaN      NA    Inf   -Inf   Inf
combined.cd   0.3300  0.3301  0.184 -0.028 0.694

Confidence level= 0.95
```

The combined results from this summary are on the log scale, and we transform back to the OR as follows:

```
> # Use `exp' function to transform back
> exp(summary(MI.exactLiuOR)$mms[49,])

            mean median stddev  CI.1 CI.2
combined.cd 1.39   1.39    1.2 0.972    2
```

This give the OR of 1.39 with 95% CI of (0.972, 2) which again indicates that there is no statistically significantly difference between the rosiglitazone group and the control group on MI.

We summarize the analyses using the novel *confidence distributions* approach implemented in gmeta in Figure 9.1 with the following R code chunk where we only include the CDs for studies 1, 10, 15, 30, 40 as well as the combined confidence distribution:

```
> # Plot the gmeta confidence distributions
> par(mfrow=c(1,2))
> plot(MI.exactLiuOR,  trials=c(1,10,15,30,40), option=T,
     xlim=c(-5,5),xlab="Liu et al's Exact log(OR) for MI")
> plot(MI.exactTianRD, trials=c(1,10,15,30,40), option=T,
     xlim=c(-0.04,0.04), xlab="Tian et al's Exact RD for MI")
```

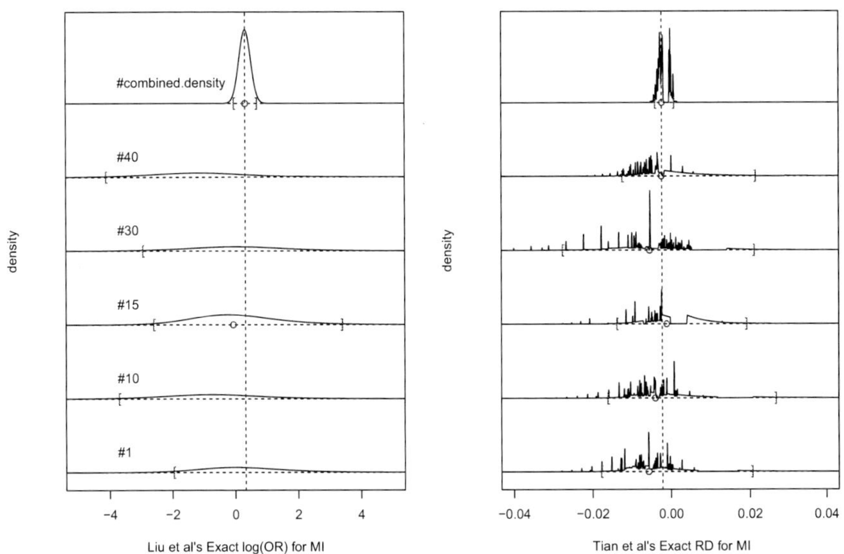

FIGURE 9.1: Confidence Distributions from Both Exact Methods

9.2.3 Data Analysis for Cardiovascular Death (Death)

Similarly we use the same steps to analyze the data for cardiovascular death (Death). We first create a dataframe only for Death as follows:

```
> datDeath    = dat[,c("Death.TRT","Death.CTRL","n.TRT","n.CTRL")]
```

For risk difference, the classical fixed-effects and random-effects meta-analysis can be performed using the following R code chunk:

```
> # Call metabin with RD=risk difference
> Death.RD.wo = metabin(Death.TRT,n.TRT,Death.CTRL,n.CTRL,
     data=datDeath,incr=0, method="Inverse", sm="RD")
> # Print the summary
> summary(Death.RD.wo)

Number of studies combined: k=48


                         RD      95%-CI   z  p.value
Fixed effect model    0.001  [0; 0.002] 2.6   0.0094
Random effects model 0.001  [0; 0.002] 2.6   0.0094


Quantifying heterogeneity:
tau^2 < 0.0001; H = 1 [1; 1]; I^2 = 0% [0%; 0%]


Test of heterogeneity:
     Q d.f. p.value
 13.69   47        1


Details on meta-analytical method:
- Inverse variance method
- DerSimonian-Laird estimator for tau^2

> # Call metabin with default setting to add 0.5
> Death.RD = metabin(Death.TRT,n.TRT,Death.CTRL,n.CTRL,
     data=datDeath, method="Inverse", sm="RD")
> # Print the summary
> summary(Death.RD)
```

```
Number of studies combined: k=48

                         RD          95%-CI     z  p.value
Fixed effect model    0.001 [-0.001;0.002] 0.943 0.3455
Random effects model 0.001 [-0.001;0.002] 0.943 0.3455

Quantifying heterogeneity:
tau^2 < 0.0001; H = 1 [1; 1]; I^2 = 0% [0%; 0%]

Test of heterogeneity:
    Q d.f. p.value
 7.92   47        1

Details on meta-analytical method:
- Inverse variance method
- DerSimonian-Laird estimator for tau^2
```

Again, we see from the summaries that the combined RD $= 0.001$ with 95% CI of (0, 0.002) and a p-value $= 0.0094$ for both fixed-effects and random-effects models without continuity correction. This statistical significance vanishes when 0.5 is added to the zero cells in 25 studies. The combined RD is now 0.001 with 95% CI of (-0.001, 0.002) and a p-value $= 0.943$ for both fixed-effects and random-effects models.

With gmeta the risk difference is implemented as follows:

```
> # Call "gmeta" with method="exact2"
> Death.exactTianRD =  gmeta(datDeath,gmi.type="2x2",
         method="exact2", ci.level=0.95,n=2000)
```

The summary for this modeling is printed as follows:

```
> summary(Death.exactTianRD)

        Exact Meta-Analysis Approach through CD-Framework

Call:
gmeta.default(gmi = datDeath, gmi.type = "2x2", method = "exact2",
```

```
    n = 2000, ci.level = 0.95)

Combined CD Summary:
               mean    median   stddev     CI.1    CI.2
exp1      -1.55e-03 -2.97e-03 0.005132 -0.01274 0.02063
exp2       1.08e-03 -1.15e-06 0.004528 -0.00749 0.01427
exp3       2.08e-03 -9.16e-07 0.005188 -0.00554 0.01723
exp4       1.81e-03 -4.80e-07 0.008317 -0.01362 0.02693
exp5      -2.94e-03 -4.31e-03 0.008163 -0.01947 0.03113
exp6       1.31e-04 -1.19e-03 0.023533       NA      NA
exp7       6.87e-05 -5.92e-07 0.008521 -0.02292 0.02371
exp8      -6.73e-03 -1.45e-02 0.026914       NA      NA
exp9       4.45e-05  3.23e-05 0.002701 -0.00718 0.00772
exp10      1.78e-03 -4.23e-04 0.006930 -0.01028 0.02180
exp11     -3.02e-03 -5.11e-03 0.010069 -0.01917 0.01200
exp12      2.52e-03 -3.20e-07 0.006694 -0.00725 0.02227
exp13      3.81e-03  4.10e-03 0.005403 -0.01231 0.01747
exp14      1.11e-03 -4.11e-07 0.004256 -0.00700 0.01394
exp15     -4.12e-03 -5.03e-03 0.005708 -0.01607 0.01830
exp16      4.84e-03  5.62e-03 0.013645 -0.01808      NA
exp17      2.48e-04 -1.00e-03 0.010064 -0.02675 0.02961
exp18     -3.44e-03 -4.51e-03 0.009007 -0.02128 0.03371
exp19     -6.44e-03 -7.02e-03 0.010694 -0.03353 0.02605
exp20     -3.97e-03 -5.54e-03 0.009487 -0.02297 0.03750
exp21      1.54e-04 -3.44e-04 0.008721 -0.02279 0.02449
exp22      1.47e-04 -1.65e-04 0.006004 -0.01583 0.01705
exp23      8.78e-05 -7.53e-07 0.018110       NA      NA
exp24     -3.63e-05 -1.75e-03 0.026734       NA      NA
exp25     -9.62e-04 -1.89e-03 0.003275 -0.00815 0.01320
exp26     -4.80e-03 -1.32e-02 0.025969       NA 0.03232
exp27     -1.21e-02 -1.46e-02 0.012116       NA 0.02518
exp28     -4.21e-03 -4.17e-03 0.006489 -0.01995 0.01505
exp29      1.58e-04 -3.29e-04 0.011882 -0.03109 0.03325
exp30     -5.62e-03 -5.39e-03 0.008944 -0.02750 0.02110
exp31      1.27e-03 -9.28e-07 0.015018 -0.02465      NA
```

```
exp32        -9.40e-05 -8.58e-04 0.002395 -0.00421 0.00968
exp33        -6.91e-04 -1.52e-03 0.002826 -0.00651 0.01123
exp34         5.64e-03  4.19e-03 0.008280 -0.01679 0.02624
exp35        -3.28e-03 -3.86e-03 0.005116 -0.01577 0.01302
exp36        -7.01e-05 -1.60e-04 0.003964 -0.01086 0.01088
exp37         1.57e-03 -1.90e-04 0.006005 -0.00930 0.01914
exp38         1.51e-04 -1.95e-04 0.006493 -0.01709 0.01843
exp39         3.30e-04 -2.08e-03 0.008065 -0.01239 0.02494
exp40        -6.02e-04 -2.33e-03 0.007125 -0.01233 0.02149
exp41        -8.61e-04 -9.91e-04 0.001884 -0.00499 0.00301
exp42         1.71e-04  1.26e-04 0.001499 -0.00377 0.00351
exp43         8.82e-04 -3.89e-07 0.018000 -0.02815      NA
exp44         1.87e-03 -1.20e-04 0.008131 -0.01253 0.02555
exp45        -3.66e-04 -5.37e-04 0.014531       NA      NA
exp46        -3.34e-04 -4.23e-03 0.042551       NA      NA
exp47         1.23e-04 -5.15e-07 0.005314 -0.01412 0.01515
exp48         1.43e-03 -6.97e-06 0.004238 -0.00507 0.01388
combined.cd -7.59e-04 -8.93e-04 0.000622 -0.00233 0.00135

Confidence level= 0.95
```

The last row contained the combined estimates and is produced as follows:

```
> summary(Death.exactTianRD)$mms[49,]

                 mean    median   stddev     CI.1    CI.2
combined.cd -0.000759 -0.000893 0.000622 -0.00233 0.00135
```

We see that the mean difference is -0.000759 with 95% CI of (-0.00233, 0.00135) indicating no statistically significant difference between rosiglitazone group and the control group on cardiovascular death.

Similarly for the odds ratio, the classical fixed-effects and random-effects models are implemented as follows:

```
> # Call metabin without 0.5 correction
> Death.OR.wo = metabin(Death.TRT,n.TRT,Death.CTRL,n.CTRL,
     data=datDeath,incr=0,method="Inverse", sm="OR")
```

```
> # Summary
> summary(Death.OR.wo)

Number of studies combined: k=23

                        OR           95%-CI     z  p.value
Fixed effect model     1.2  [0.642; 2.24] 0.568   0.5699
Random effects model 1.2  [0.642; 2.24] 0.568   0.5699

Quantifying heterogeneity:
tau^2 < 0.0001; H = 1 [1; 1]; I^2 = 0% [0%; 0%]

Test of heterogeneity:
    Q d.f. p.value
 1.02   22       1

Details on meta-analytical method:
- Inverse variance method
- DerSimonian-Laird estimator for tau^2

> # Call metabin with default 0.5 correction
> Death.OR = metabin(Death.TRT,n.TRT,Death.CTRL,n.CTRL,
     data=datDeath, method="Inverse", sm="OR")
> # Print the Summary
> summary(Death.OR)

Number of studies combined: k=23

                        OR           95%-CI     z  p.value
Fixed effect model    1.31  [0.805; 2.13] 1.08   0.2783
Random effects model 1.31  [0.805; 2.13] 1.08   0.2783

Quantifying heterogeneity:
tau^2 < 0.0001; H = 1 [1; 1]; I^2 = 0% [0%; 0%]

Test of heterogeneity:
```

```
   Q d.f. p.value
 4.79   22       1

Details on meta-analytical method:
- Inverse variance method
- DerSimonian-Laird estimator for tau^2
```

We see that with or without the default 0.5 continuity correction, the 95% CIs and p-values are slightly different, but yield the same conclusion that there is no statistically significant difference between the rosiglitazone group and the control group on cardiovascular death.

Now we call `gmeta` for the exact method for the odds ratio which is implemented as follows:

```
> # Call "gmeta" for "exact1" on OR
> Death.exactLiuOR  =  gmeta(datDeath,gmi.type="2x2",
         method="exact1", ci.level=0.95,n=2000)
> # Print the summary
> summary(Death.exactLiuOR)

                Exact Meta-Analysis Approach through CD-Framework


Call:
gmeta.default(gmi = datDeath, gmi.type = "2x2", method = "exact1",
   n = 2000, ci.level = 0.95)


Combined CD Summary:
                mean median stddev   CI.1 CI.2
exp1             Inf     NA    Inf -3.651  Inf
exp2             NaN     NA    Inf   -Inf  Inf
exp3             NaN     NA    Inf   -Inf  Inf
exp4             NaN     NA    Inf   -Inf  Inf
exp5             Inf     NA    Inf -3.636  Inf
exp6             NaN     NA    Inf   -Inf  Inf
exp7             NaN     NA    Inf   -Inf  Inf
exp8           0.461  0.426  0.979 -1.473 2.59
```

```
exp9         NaN    NA   Inf   -Inf  Inf
exp10        NaN    NA   Inf   -Inf  Inf
exp11      0.779 0.661 1.360 -1.859 4.11
exp12        NaN    NA   Inf   -Inf  Inf
exp13       -Inf    NA   Inf   -Inf 2.95
exp14        NaN    NA   Inf   -Inf  Inf
exp15        Inf    NA   Inf -1.934  Inf
exp16     -0.651 -0.652 1.634 -4.320 3.02
exp17        NaN    NA   Inf   -Inf  Inf
exp18        Inf    NA   Inf -3.627  Inf
exp19        Inf    NA   Inf -2.937  Inf
exp20        Inf    NA   Inf -3.657  Inf
exp21        NaN    NA   Inf   -Inf  Inf
exp22        NaN    NA   Inf   -Inf  Inf
exp23        NaN    NA   Inf   -Inf  Inf
exp24        NaN    NA   Inf   -Inf  Inf
exp25        Inf    NA   Inf -3.653  Inf
exp26      0.712 0.594 1.365 -1.934 4.05
exp27        Inf    NA   Inf -1.278  Inf
exp28        Inf    NA   Inf -2.898  Inf
exp29        NaN    NA   Inf   -Inf  Inf
exp30        Inf    NA   Inf -2.921  Inf
exp31        NaN    NA   Inf   -Inf  Inf
exp32        Inf    NA   Inf -4.084  Inf
exp33        Inf    NA   Inf -3.719  Inf
exp34       -Inf    NA   Inf   -Inf 2.85
exp35        Inf    NA   Inf -2.973  Inf
exp36        NaN    NA   Inf   -Inf  Inf
exp37        NaN    NA   Inf   -Inf  Inf
exp38        NaN    NA   Inf   -Inf  Inf
exp39        Inf    NA   Inf -4.306  Inf
exp40        Inf    NA   Inf -4.107  Inf
exp41      0.183 0.180 0.435 -0.672 1.05
exp42     -0.246 -0.186 0.877 -2.235 1.40
exp43        NaN    NA   Inf   -Inf  Inf
```

```
exp44          NaN     NA    Inf    -Inf  Inf
exp45          NaN     NA    Inf    -Inf  Inf
exp46          NaN     NA    Inf    -Inf  Inf
exp47          NaN     NA    Inf    -Inf  Inf
exp48          NaN     NA    Inf    -Inf  Inf
combined.cd  0.385  0.385  0.343 -0.268 1.09

Confidence level= 0.95
```

The combined results from this summary are on the log scale. We transform back to the OR as follows:

```
> exp(summary(Death.exactLiuOR)$mms[49,])

              mean median stddev  CI.1 CI.2
combined.cd 1.47    1.47   1.41 0.765 2.97
```

This gives an OR of 1.47 with 95% CI of (0.765, 2.97), which again indicates that there is no statistically significant difference between the rosiglitazone group and the control group on cardiovascular death. A figure similar to Figure 9.1 can be produced and we leave this as an exercise for interested readers.

9.3 Discussion

In this chapter, we discussed meta-analysis of rare events based upon the well-known rosiglitazone dataset using the novel *confidence distribution* approach developed to unify the framework of meta-analysis. We pointed out that the classical fixed-effects and random-effects models are not appropriate for rare events. We recommend the new *confidence distribution* procedure which can combine test results based on exact distributions. The application of this new procedure is made easy with the R package `gmeta`.

For further reading, we recommend Sutton et al. (2002) which provides a review of meta-analyses for rare and adverse event data from the aspects of model choice, continuity corrections, exact statistics, Bayesian methods and sensitivity analysis. There are other newly developed methods for meta-analysis of rare-events. Cai et al. (2010) proposed some approaches based on Poisson random-effects models for statistical inference about the relative risk between two treatment groups. To develop fixed-effects and random-effects moment-based meta-analytic methods to analyze binary adverse-event data, Bhaumik et al. (2012) derived three new methods which include a simple (unweighted) average treatment effect estimator, a new heterogeneity estimator, and a parametric bootstrapping test for heterogeneity. Readers may explore these methods for other applications.

Chapter 10

Other R Packages for Meta-Analysis

There are many R packages for meta-analysis and we have so far illustrated three commonly-used ones: `rmeta` by Lumley (2009), `meta` by Schwarzer (2010) and `metafor` by Viechtbauer (2010), in the previous chapters. As seen from the illustration in the previous chapter, all three packages can serve as "general purpose" packages for arbitrary effect-size and different outcome measures to fit fixed-effects and random-effects meta-analysis models. From our experience, all three packages are easy to use for meta-analysis with `metafor` having more methods implemented. For example in random-effect meta-analysis, `rmeta` only implemented the DerSimonian-Laird estimator to estimate the between-study variance of τ^2 where `metafor` and `meta` included several other methods, such as the restricted maximum-likelihood estimator, the maximum-likelihood estimator, the Hunter-Schmidt estimator, the Sidik-Jonkman estimator, the Hedges estimator, and the Empirical Bayes estimator. In addition, `metafor` has a great feature for meta-regression as illustrated in Chapter 7 and can be used to include multiple continuous or categorical regression covariates as well as mixed-effects models, whereas `meta` can only include a single categorical regression covariate in fixed-effects, and no meta-regression is included in `rmeta`. A comprehensive comparison and discussion of these three packages can be found in Table 2 of Viechtbauer (2010).

In this chapter, we introduce and illustrate some extra R functions and packages designed for specific meta-analysis and provide discussion for listing more R packages for further reference. Readers can search the R homepage for packages for their own research and applications. Specifically, we present methods to combine p-values from studies in Section 10.1. In Section 10.2, we introduce several R packages for meta-analysis of correlation coefficients and illustrate their applications to a real dataset on land use intensity across 18 gradients from nine countries. Multivariate meta-analysis is presented in Section 10.3 with a real dataset using the R package `mvmeta` followed by discussion in Section 10.4 to introduce additional R packages for specific meta-analysis.

10.1 Combining p-Values in Meta-Analysis

When summarizing a study for statistical purposes, a p-value is usually reported. In meta-analysis to combine several independent studies with reported p-values, we can combine the p-values to obtain an overall p-value.

There are several methods for combining p-values; see for example in Hartung et al. (2008) and Peace (1991). The most commonly used one is Fisher's method. There is no need for a R package for this calculation since it is very straightforward to write a simple R code for this purpose.

Fisher's method is known as Fisher's combined probability test which was developed to combine statistical p-values from several independent tests of the same hypothesis (H_0) using a χ^2-distribution. Specifically, suppose p_i is the p-value reported from ith study, then the statistic

$$X^2 = -2\sum_{i=1}^{K} ln(p_i) \tag{10.1}$$

is distributed as χ^2-distribution with $2K$-degrees of freedom - since under the null hypothesis for test i, its p-value p_i follows a uniform distribution on the interval [0,1], i.e. $p_i \sim U[0,1]$. By taking the negative natural logarithm of a uniformly distributed value, $-ln(p_i)$ follows an exponential distribution. Multiplying this exponentially distributed statistic by a factor of two produces a χ^2-distributed quantity of $-2ln(p_i)$ with two degrees of freedom. The sum of K independent χ^2, each with two degrees of freedom , follows a χ^2 distribution with $2K$ degrees of freedom. Intuitively we can see that if the p_i are small, the test statistic X^2 would be large, suggesting that the null hypothesis is not true for the combined test.

Based on this formulation, we can write a R function for Fisher's method as follows:

```
> # Create a function for Fisher's method
```

```
> fishers.pvalue = function(x){
 # Call chisq prob function for calculation
 pchisq(-2 * sum(log(x)),df=2*length(x),lower=FALSE)
 }
```

In this R function, x is the vector of p-values from all independent studies.

As an example, we make use of the data in Table 4.1 for Coronary Death or MI of Statin Use. In Section 4.2.1.2, we calculated the p-values for the 4 studies to compare the experimental to standard groups and the values are 0.106, 0.0957, 0.00166 and 0.0694, respectively. The following R code chunk illustrates the application of Fisher's method:

```
> # The reported p-values
> x = c(0.106, 0.0957, 0.00166, 0.0694)
> # Call function of fishers.pvalue
> combined.pval = fishers.pvalue(x)
> print(combined.pval)
```

```
[1] 0.000623
```

This gives a combined p-value of 0.00062 indicating strong statistical significance overall. A proper interpretation of this result is: When the four studies are taken as an aggregate, Fisher's method for combining p-values provides evidence that intensive statin therapy is more effective than standard statin therapy in reducing the risk of myocardial infarction or cardiac death.

10.2 R Packages for Meta-Analysis of Correlation Coefficients

There are several packages for meta-analysis of correlation coefficients. The R package of `meta` and `metafor` introduced above can be used to combine correlation coefficients from studies. We illustrate another package of `metacor` in this section for this purpose along with discussion for an additional R package `MAc`.

10.2.1 Introduction

Package `metafor` is designed for meta-analysis of correlation coefficients and is maintained by Etienne Laliberte (etiennelaliberte@gmail.com). The comprehensive information about this package can be seen from the website at `http://cran.r-project.org/web/packages/metacor/index.html` with package download and reference manual.

Readers can download the package from this webpage and load this package to the R console using:

```
> library(metacor)
```

For `help` about this package, simply use the general "help" function as follows:

```
> library(help=metafor)
```

It can be seen from this "help" function that two approaches are implemented in this package to meta-analyze correlation coefficients as effect sizes reported from studies. These two approaches are the DerSimonian-Laird (DSL) and Olkin-Pratt (OP) methods as discussed in Schulze (2004). Based on these two methods, two functions are implemented in this package as:

1. `metacor.DSL` for DerSimonian-Laird (DSL) approach with correlation coefficients as effect sizes,

2. `metacor.OP` for Olkin-Pratt (OP) approach with correlation coefficients as effect sizes.

10.2.2 Example

To illustrate the application of the approaches in this package, we make use of the data given in the package which is named as `lui`. This `lui` includes two correlation coefficients between *l*and *u*se *i*ntensity and response diversity (variable named as `r.FDis`) or functional redundancy (variable named as `r.nbsp`) along with the total observations (variable named as `n`) across 18 land use intensity gradients from nine countries and five biomes. The data can be loaded into R as follows:

```
> # Load the data into R
> data(lui)
> # Print the data
> lui

                                label    r.FDis  r.nbsp   n
15                  New Zealand (TG) -4.30e-01 -0.3790  72
1               Australia / NSW (STR) -4.24e-01 -0.6042 176
4           Australia / Mungalli (TR) -3.78e-01 -0.8438  36
12             Nicaragua / Rivas (TR) -3.70e-01 -0.5482  42
5          Australia / Atherton (TR) -3.29e-01 -0.4882 315
11          Nicaragua / Matiguas (TR) -1.37e-01 -0.6163  42
2               Australia / QLD (STR) -1.16e-01 -0.3791 117
14               Australia / NSW (TW) -1.08e-01 -0.0841 332
16                      Portugal (TF) -4.58e-02 -0.0513 120
3              Australia / Tully (TR)  2.29e-17  0.1010  80
6        Costa Rica / Las Cruces (TR)  1.54e-02 -0.0400 297
17               Canada / Quebec (TF)  2.46e-02  0.0160 240
8         Costa Rica / La Palma (TR)  4.06e-02  0.0161 290
18         USA / North Carolina (TF)  1.11e-01 -0.4326  26
13                          Laos (TR)  1.35e-01  0.0239  96
10       China / Hainan montane (TR)  1.39e-01 -0.1453  36
9        China / Hainan lowland (TR)  1.71e-01 -0.3880  48
7   Costa Rica / Puerto Jimenez (TR)  2.01e-01  0.1213 290
```

Meta-analysis for `r.FDis` is performed in the package as an example and we illustrate these two approaches for `r.nbsp`. The DerSimonian-Laird (DSL) approach meta-analysis can be performed with R code chunk as follows:

```
> # Call metacor.DSL for DerSimonian-Laird (DSL) approach
> nbsp.DSL.metacor = metacor.DSL(lui$r.nbsp, lui$n, lui$label)
> # Print the result
> nbsp.DSL.metacor

$z
 [1] -0.3988 -0.6997 -1.2343 -0.6158 -0.5337 -0.7190
 [7] -0.3990 -0.0843 -0.0513  0.1013 -0.0400  0.0160
```

```
[13]  0.0161 -0.4631  0.0239 -0.1463 -0.4094  0.1219
$z.var
 [1] 0.01449 0.00578 0.03030 0.02564 0.00321 0.02564
 [7] 0.00877 0.00304 0.00855 0.01299 0.00340 0.00422
[13] 0.00348 0.04348 0.01075 0.03030 0.02222 0.00348
$z.lower
 [1] -0.1629 -0.5506 -0.8932 -0.3020 -0.4227 -0.4051
 [7] -0.2155  0.0238  0.1299  0.3247  0.0743  0.1433
[13]  0.1318 -0.0545  0.2272  0.1949 -0.1172  0.2376
$r.lower
 [1] -0.1615 -0.5010 -0.7129 -0.2931 -0.3992 -0.3843
 [7] -0.2122  0.0238  0.1292  0.3137  0.0742  0.1423
[13]  0.1310 -0.0544  0.2233  0.1925 -0.1167  0.2332
$z.upper
 [1] -0.63479 -0.84867 -1.57553 -0.92967 -0.64462 -1.03281
 [7] -0.58261 -0.19236 -0.23252 -0.12203 -0.15431 -0.11134
[13] -0.09961 -0.87181 -0.17932 -0.48749 -0.70156  0.00617
$r.upper
 [1] -0.56134 -0.69038 -0.91790 -0.73044 -0.56804 -0.77503
 [7] -0.52456 -0.19002 -0.22842 -0.12143 -0.15310 -0.11089
[13] -0.09928 -0.70229 -0.17742 -0.45222 -0.60536  0.00617
$z.mean
[1] -0.286
$r.mean
[1] -0.278
$z.mean.se
[1] 0.0742
$z.mean.lower
[1] -0.14
$r.mean.lower
[1] -0.14
$z.mean.upper
[1] -0.431
$r.mean.upper
[1] -0.407
```

```
$p
[1] 5.85e-05
```

The first part of the results reports the study-specific z-values, the variances of each z, the lower/upper limits of the confidence intervals for each z and the lower/upper limits of the confidence intervals for each r. The second part of the results reflects the combined results from the meta-analysis. From the study-specific confidence intervals, we can see that some studies have significant correlation coefficients and some do not. However, when combined, the correlation coefficient is -0.278 with lower CI bound of -0.14 and upper bound of -0.407. The p-value from the z-test is 0 which indicates significant correlation for the studies combined. The default setting in `metacor.DSL` provides the forest plot which is given by Figure 10.1.

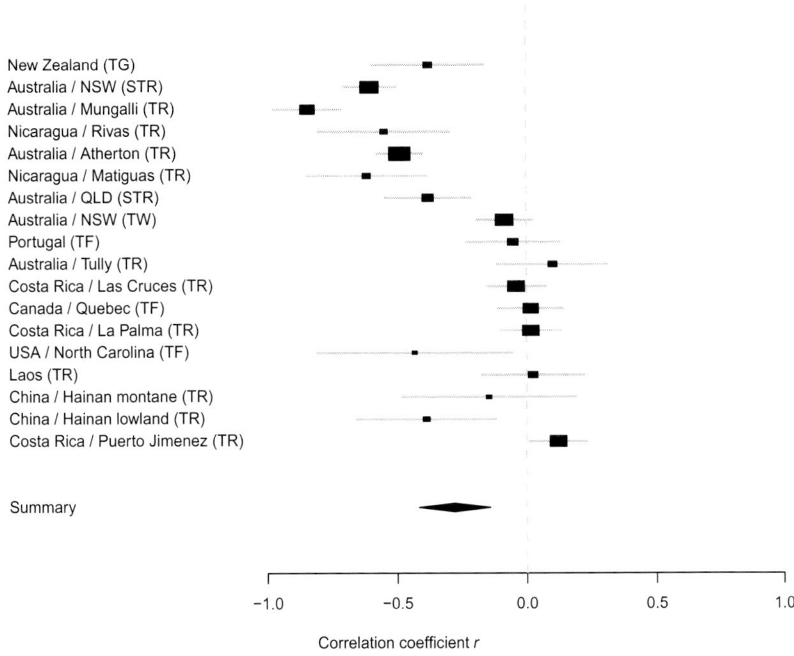

FIGURE 10.1: Meta-Analysis for Correlation Coefficients of *nbsp*

Similar analysis can be performed for the Olkin-Pratt (OP) approach. But we do not make the forest plot here; rather we specify the `plot=F` (note that the `plot=T` is the default setting to generate the forest plot). Instead of printing all the results, we only print the p-value for the meta-analysis result to save space. The R code chunk is as follows:

```
> # Call metacor.OP for Olkin-Pratt (OP) approach
> nbsp.OP.metacor=metacor.OP(lui$r.nbsp,lui$n,lui$label,plot=F)
> # Print the p-value only
> nbsp.OP.metacor$p
```

```
[1] 1.11e-18
```

The same type of meta-analysis can be done by using the `metacor` function from R package `meta` with the following R code chunk; we print only the summary results without the individual-study data:

```
> # Load the library
> library(meta)
> # Call metacor for meta-analysis
> nbsp.DSLfromMeta=metacor(cor=r.nbsp,n=n,studlab=label,data=lui)
> # Print the summary result
> summary(nbsp.DSLfromMeta)
```

```
Number of studies combined: k=18

                         COR            95%-CI     z  p.value
Fixed effect model    -0.182 [-0.219;-0.145] -9.40 <0.0001
Random effects model -0.278 [-0.407;-0.140] -3.85  0.0001

Quantifying heterogeneity:
tau^2 = 0.0861; H = 3.61 [3.06; 4.25]; I^2 = 92.3% [89.3%; 94.5%]

Test of heterogeneity:
     Q d.f.  p.value
 221.1   17 < 0.0001
```

```
Details on meta-analytical method:
- Inverse variance method
- DerSimonian-Laird estimator for tau^2
- Fisher's z transformation of correlations
```

Comparing these summary results (just the part of the random-effects model) with those from `nbsp.DSL.metacort`,we note that they are the same. Readers can call functions `escalc` and `rma` from R package `metafor` to reproduce the results. Notice that `meta` and `metafor` have more options to perform meta-analysis for correlation coefficients.

10.2.3 Discussion

R package `MAc` (Meta-Analysis for Correlations) can also be used to combine correlation coefficients. This package can be obtained from `http://rwiki.sciviews.org/doku.php?id=packages:cran:ma_meta-analysis`. The authors implemented the recommended procedures as described in Cooper et al. (2009). Including package `MAc`, there are in fact five related packages from this site which are `MAc GUI`, `MAd` (Meta-Analysis for Differences), `MAd GUI` and `compute.es`. Note that `compute.es` is a package to convert and standardize various within-study effect-sizes and calculate the associated variances for further meta-analysis. The packages `MAc` and `MAc GUI` are the packages for meta-analysis of correlation coefficients with `MAc GUI` as the graphical user interface (GUI) version of `MAc`.

Because of this graphical user interface (GUI), this package suite can integrate the meta-analytical approaches to achieve a user-friendly graphical user interface (GUI) so that meta-analysis can be performed in a menu-driven (i.e. "point and click") fashion for readers who are not versed in coding. Examples and illustrations can be found from the webpage.

10.3 Multivariate Meta-Analysis

It is not uncommon for studies to produce multiple outcome measures which leads to statistical multivariate analysis. For example, the dataset `lui` in Section 10.2 contains two correlation coefficients between *l*and *u*se *i*ntensity and response diversity (variable named as `r.FDis`) or functional redundancy (variable named as `r.nbsp`) along with the total observations (variable named as `n`) across 18 land use intensity gradients from nine countries and five biomes. It is easy to find more examples in multivariate meta-analysis. It is noted that multivariate meta-analysis is simply an extension of the univariate meta-analysis with multiple outcome measures where the correlations among the multiple outcomes have to be taken into account. With study-level moderators or predictors, multivariate meta-regression can be also developed in parallel with multivariate regression techniques.

In this section, we introduce multivariate meta-analysis using the R package `mvmeta` as detailed in Gasparrini and Kenward (2012). This package includes a collection of functions to perform fixed- and random-effects multivariate meta-analysis along with univariate meta-analysis as well as meta-regression.

10.3.1 The Model and the Package of `mvmeta`

Suppose that there are M outcomes $\mathbf{y_i} = (y_{1i}, y_{2i}, \cdots, y_{Mi})$ reported from K studies where $\mathbf{y_i}$ is the vector of M outcomes of y_{mi} from the mth outcome and ith study $(i = 1, \cdots, K)$ For p-study level moderators or predictors, the general multivariate meta-regression model is formulated as follows:

$$\mathbf{y_i} \sim N_M(\mathbf{X_i}\beta, \mathbf{S_i} + \Psi) \tag{10.2}$$

where $\mathbf{y_i}$ is distributed as multivariate normal with mean $\mathbf{X_i}\beta$ and variance-covariance matrix of $\mathbf{S_i} + \Psi$. In this formulation,$\mathbf{X_i}$ is a $K \times Kp$ design matrix and β is the vector of fixed-effects coefficients. $\mathbf{S_i}$ is the within covariance matrix from the M outcomes which is assumed known. Ψ is the so-called between-study covariance matrix which is assumed to be zero for fixed-effects meta-models, but estimated from the data in random-effects meta-models.

It can be easily seen that when p=1, the general meta-regression model 10.2 becomes the meta-analysis model where $\mathbf{X_i}$ reduces to an identity matrix and β reduces to the intercepts. When $K = 1$, this model reduces to the corresponding univariate meta-regression or meta-analysis model.

Therefore the purpose is to estimate and make statistical inference for the coefficients β and, for random-effects models, estimate the between-study covariance matrix Ψ as seen in equation 10.2. The R package `mvmeta` is developed for this purpose.

This R package can be accessed from `http://cran.r-project.org/web/packages/mvmeta/index.html`. The reference manual is in the pdf file `mvmeta.pdf`. With this package installed in R, the reader can access its help manual using `library(help=mvmeta)`. We use some examples from this package in this chapter to further promote and illustrate its functionalities.

10.3.2 Examples

When the package is installed in R, it can accessed by calling this library as follows:

```
> library(mvmeta)
```

There are several examples in the package. We illustrate this package using data `berkey98` which includes five published clinical trials on periodontal disease as reported in Berkey et al. (1995) and Berkey et al. (1998). This dataset is loaded into R as follows:

```
> # Load the Data
> data(berkey98)
> # Print the data
> berkey98
```

```
          pubyear npat   PD    AL var_PD cov_PD_AL var_AL
Pihlstrom    1983   14 0.47 -0.32 0.0075    0.0030 0.0077
Lindhe       1982   15 0.20 -0.60 0.0057    0.0009 0.0008
Knowles      1979   78 0.40 -0.12 0.0021    0.0007 0.0014
Ramfjord     1987   89 0.26 -0.31 0.0029    0.0009 0.0015
Becker       1988   16 0.56 -0.39 0.0148    0.0072 0.0304
```

It can be seen that this dataset includes five published studies that compare surgical and non-surgical treatments for medium-severity periodontal disease. The two outcome measures are average improvement (surgical minus non-surgical, in mm) in probing depth (PD) and attachment level (AL). In this dataframe, 7 variables are reported with `pubyear` as the publication year of the trial, `npat` as the number of patients in each trial, `PD` as the estimated improvement from surgical to non-surgical treatment in probing depth (mm), `AL` as the estimated improvement from surgical to non-surgical treatment in attachment level (mm), `var_PD` as the variance for `PD`, `cov_PD_AL` as the co-variance between `PD` and `AL` and `var_AL` as the variance for `AL`.

The fixed-effects meta-analysis is implemented using `method="fixed"` as follows:

```
> # Call mvmeta with fixed-effects
> berkey.meta.fixed = mvmeta(cbind(PD,AL),
          S=berkey98[,c("var_PD","cov_PD_AL","var_AL")],
            method="fixed",data=berkey98)
> # Print the summary
> summary(berkey.meta.fixed)
```

```
Call: mvmeta(formula=cbind(PD,AL)~1,S=berkey98[, c("var_PD",
   "cov_PD_AL","var_AL")],data=berkey98, method = "fixed")

Multivariate fixed-effects meta-analysis
Dimension: 2

Fixed-effects coefficients
  Estimate Std.Error        z Pr(>|z|) 95%ci.lb 95%ci.ub
PD  0.3072    0.0286   0.7513   0.0000   0.2512   0.3632  ***
AL -0.3944    0.0186 -21.1471   0.0000  -0.4309  -0.3578  ***
---
Signif. codes:  0 `***' 0.001 `**' 0.01 `*' 0.05 `.' 0.1 ` ' 1

Multivariate Cochran Q-test for heterogeneity:
Q = 128.2267 (df = 8), p-value = 0.0000
I-square statistic = 93.8%
```

```
5 studies,10 observations,2 fixed and 0 random-effects params
  logLik        AIC        BIC
-45.4416   94.8833   95.4884
```

From the output we note that both PD and AL are statistically significant with estimates of effects of 0.3072 and -0.3944 for PD and AL, respectively. And there is statistically significant heterogeneity as reported by the `Multivariate Cochran Q-test for heterogeneity` with $Q = 128.2267$ (df = 8) which gives a p-value = 0.0000.

The random-effects meta-model with default method of "REML" is illustrated as follows:

```
> berkey.meta.REML = mvmeta(cbind(PD,AL), method="reml",
   S=berkey98[,c("var_PD","cov_PD_AL","var_AL")],data=berkey98)
> #Print the summary
> summary(berkey.meta.REML)

Call:mvmeta(formula=cbind(PD,AL)~1,S=berkey98[, c("var_PD",
    "cov_PD_AL", "var_AL")], data = berkey98, method = "reml")

Multivariate random-effects meta-analysis
Dimension: 2
Estimation method: REML
Variance-covariance matrix Psi: unstructured

Fixed-effects coefficients
  Estimate Std.Error     z  Pr(>|z|) 95%ci.lb 95%ci.ub
PD  0.3534    0.0588  6.0057 0.0000  0.2381    0.4688 ***
AL -0.3392    0.0879 -3.8589 0.0001 -0.5115   -0.1669 ***

Variance components:between-studies Std.Dev and correlation
    Std. Dev       PD       AL
PD    0.1083   1.0000        .
AL    0.1807   0.6088   1.0000
```

```
Multivariate Cochran Q-test for heterogeneity:
Q = 128.2267 (df = 8), p-value = 0.0000
I-square statistic = 93.8%

5 studies,10 observations,2 fixed and 3 random-effects params
logLik     AIC     BIC
2.0823  5.8353  6.2325
```

Again both PD and AL are statistically significant with estimates of effects of 0.3534 and -0.3392 for PD and AL, respectively,with the same conclusion for the test of heterogeneity. For the random-effects meta-model, the estimated between-studies standard deviations are $\hat{\tau}_{PD} = 0.1083$ and $\hat{\tau}_{AL} = 0.1807$ with estimated correlation of 0.6088.

Slightly different estimates (but the same statistical conclusions) will result if the maximum likelihood method is used as seen from the following R code chunk:

```
> berkey.meta.ML = mvmeta(cbind(PD,AL),
     S=berkey98[,c("var_PD","cov_PD_AL","var_AL")],
     method="ml",data=berkey98)
> summary(berkey.meta.ML)

Call:mvmeta(formula=cbind(PD,AL)~1,S=berkey98[,c("var_PD",
    "cov_PD_AL", "var_AL")], data = berkey98, method = "ml")

Multivariate random-effects meta-analysis
Dimension: 2
Estimation method: ML
Variance-covariance matrix Psi: unstructured

Fixed-effects coefficients
  Estimate Std.Error       z  Pr(>|z|) 95%ci.lb 95%ci.ub
PD  0.3448    0.0495  6.9714 0.0000    0.2479    0.4418 ***
AL -0.3379    0.0798 -4.2365 0.0000   -0.4943   -0.1816 ***

Variance components:between-studies Std. Dev and correlation
```

```
    Std. Dev       PD       AL
PD    0.0837   1.0000        .
AL    0.1617   0.6992   1.0000

Multivariate Cochran Q-test for heterogeneity:
Q = 128.2267 (df = 8), p-value = 0.0000
I-square statistic = 93.8%

5 studies,10 observations,2 fixed and 3 random-effects params
 logLik       AIC       BIC
 5.8407   -1.6813   -0.1684
```

To account for between-study heterogeneity, we use study-level moderators, which in this dataset is the year of the clinical trial as `studyyear`. The implementation is straightforward and we only show the random-effects meta-regression with "REML". Interested readers can experiment using the `method="fixed"` and `method="ml"`.

The R code chunk is as follows:

```
> # meta-reg to study year
> berkey.metareg.REML = mvmeta(cbind(PD,AL)~pubyear,
  S=berkey98[,c("var_PD","cov_PD_AL","var_AL")],data=berkey98)
> # Print the result
> summary(berkey.metareg.REML)

Call:mvmeta(formula=cbind(PD,AL)~pubyear,S=berkey98[,c("var_PD",
    "cov_PD_AL", "var_AL")], data = berkey98)

Multivariate random-effects meta-regression
Dimension: 2
Estimation method: REML
Variance-covariance matrix Psi: unstructured

Fixed-effects coefficients
PD :
          Estimate Std.Error    z  Pr(>|z|) 95%ci.lb 95%ci.ub
```

```
(Intercept) -9.281   43.341  -0.214  0.830  -94.230  75.666
pubyear      0.004    0.021   0.222  0.823   -0.038   0.047

             Estimate Std.Error     z  Pr(>|z|) 95%ci.lb  95%ci.ub
(Intercept) 22.541    59.430  0.379   0.704  -93.940   139.023
pubyear     -0.011     0.030 -0.385   0.700   -0.070     0.047
---
Signif. codes:  0 `***' 0.001 `**' 0.01 `*' 0.05 `.' 0.1 ` ' 1

Variance components:between-studies Std. Dev and correlation
    Std. Dev      PD       AL
PD    0.1430  1.0000        .
AL    0.2021  0.5614  1.0000

Multivariate Cochran Q-test for residual heterogeneity:
Q = 125.7557 (df = 6), p-value = 0.0000
I-square statistic = 95.2%

5 studies,10 observations,4 fixed and 3 random-effects params
 logLik      AIC      BIC
-3.5400  21.0799  19.6222
```

It can be seen from the summary that the moderator is not statistically significant for any PD (p-value=0.8239) and AL (p-value= 0.7002). Because of this non-significance, the Cochran heterogeneity statistic Q changed slightly from 128.2267 in the meta-model to 125.7557 in the meta-regression.

10.3.3 Summary

In this section, we further illustrated features of the package `mvmeta` for multivariate meta-analysis. This package can also be used for meta-regression to incorporate study-level moderators and predictors. To promote application of the package, we illustrated its use with an example for both fixed-effects and random-effects models.

There are more packages that can be used for multivariate meta-analysis. For example, `mvtmeta` is another R package for multivariate meta-analysis developed by Chen et al. (2012). It can be accessed from `http://cran.r-project.org/web/packages/mvtmeta/index.html`. This package contains two functions `mvtmeta_fe` for fixed-effects multivariate meta-analysis and `mvtmeta_re` for random-effects multivariate meta-analysis which are easy to implement.

Another function that can be used for multivariate meta-analysis is from the genetic analysis package, i.e. `gap`, which can be accessed at `http://cran.r-project.org/web/packages/gap/`. This package is in fact designed to be an integrated package for genetic data analysis of both population and family data. The function `mvmeta` can be used for multivariate meta-analysis based on generalized least squares. This function can input a data matrix of parameter estimates (denoted by b) and their variance-covariance matrix from individual studies (denoted by V) and output a generalized least squares (GLS) estimate and heterogeneity statistic. The usage is `mvmeta(b,V)`. An example is given in the package for readers to follow.

For a Bayesian approach to multivariate meta-analysis, `DPpackage` is a good reference and can be obtained from `http://cran.r-project.org/web/packages/DPpackage/`. This package contains functions to provide inference via simulation from the posterior distributions for Bayesian nonparametric and semiparametric models which is motivated by the Dirichlet Process prior so named as `DPpackage`. In this package, the function `DPmultmeta` is used for Bayesian analysis in semiparametric random-effects multivariate meta-analysis model.

10.4 Discussion

There are many more R packages available from the R website. Searching "R Site Search" for "meta-analysis" produces several additional packages. We recommend interested readers to search for packages for their own applications if the packages introduced in this book are insufficient.

We mention a few more packages for further reference and to promote the use of these packages to conclude the book.

1. `metaMA` is a package developed by Guillemette Marot for "Meta-Analysis for Microarray" (Marot et al., 2009) and is available at `http://cran.r-project.org/web/packages/metaMA/`. This package combines either p-values or modified effect-sizes from different microarray studies to find differentially expressed genes.

2. `MAMA`, developed by Ivana Ihnatova, is a similar package for "Meta-Analysis for Microarray" and is available at `http://cran.r-project.org/web/packages/MAMA/`. A very detailed description of this package can be found at `http://cran.r-project.org/web/packages/MAMA/vignettes/MAMA.pdf` where the descriptions of nine different methods are implemented for meta-analysis of microarray studies.

3. `MetaDE`, developed by Xingbin Wang, Jia Li and George C. Tseng, is another R package for microarray meta-analysis for differentially expressed gene detection and is available at `http://cran.r-project.org/web/packages/MetaDE/`. The reference manual can be found from `http://cran.r-project.org/web/packages/MetaDE/MetaDE.pdf` and describes the implementation of 12 major meta-analysis methods for differential gene expression analysis.

4. `mada`, developed by Philipp Doebler, is a package for meta-analysis of diagnostic accuracy and ROC curves and is available at `http://cran.r-project.org/web/packages/mada/`. A very detailed description of this package can be found at `http://cran.r-project.org/web/packages/mada/vignettes/mada.pdf`. As described in the file, this package "provides some established and some current approaches to diagnostic meta-analysis, as well as functions to produce descriptive statistics and graphics. It is hopefully complete enough to be the only tool needed for a diagnostic meta-analysis."

5. `HSROC`, created by Ian Schiller and Nandini Dendukuri, is a package for joint meta-analysis of diagnostic test sensitivity and specificity with or without a gold standard reference test. This package is available at `http://cran.r-project.org/web/packages/HSROC/` and "implements a model for joint meta-analysis of sensitivity and specificity of the diagnostic test under evaluation, while taking into account the possibly

imperfect sensitivity and specificity of the reference test. This hierarchical model accounts for both within and between study variability. Estimation is carried out using a Bayesian approach, implemented via a Gibbs sampler. The model can be applied in situations where more than one reference test is used in the selected studies."

6. `bamdit`, created by Pablo Emilio Verde and Arnold Sykosch, is a package for Bayesian meta-analysis of diagnostic test data based on a scale mixtures bivariate random-effects model. This package is available at `http://cran.r-project.org/web/packages/bamdit/`.

7. `MetaPCA`, created by Don Kang and George Tseng, is a package for meta-analysis in dimension reduction of genomic data and is available at `http://cran.r-project.org/web/packages/MetaPCA/` or `https://github.com/donkang75/MetaPCA`. This package contains functions for simultaneous dimension reduction using PCA when multiple studies are combined. Two basic ideas are implemented for finding a common PC subspace by eigenvalue maximization approach and angle minimization approach, as well as incorporating Robust PCA and Sparse PCA in the meta-analysis realm.

8. `gemtc`, developed by Gert van Valkenhoef and Joel Kuiper, is a package for network meta-analysis and is available at `http://cran.r-project.org/web/packages/gemtc/` or `http://drugis.org/gemtc`. As described in this package, network meta-analysis, known as mixed treatment comparison (MTC), "is a technique to meta-analyze networks of trials comparing two or more treatments at the same time. Using a Bayesian hierarchical model, all direct and indirect comparisons are taken into account to arrive at a single, integrated, estimate of the effect of all included treatments based on all included studies."

9. `ipdmeta`, developed by S. Kovalchik, is a package for subgroup analyses with multiple trial data using aggregate statistics and is available at `http://cran.r-project.org/web/packages/ipdmeta/`. This package provides functions for an IPD linear mixed effects model for continuous outcomes and any categorical covariate from study summary statistics.

Other functions are also provided to estimate the power of a treatment-covariate interaction test.

10. `psychometric` is a package for psychometric applications and contains functions for meta-analysis besides the typical contents for correlation theory, reliability, item analysis, inter-rater reliability, and classical utility. This package is developed by Thomas D. Fletcher and is available at `http://cran.r-project.org/web/packages/psychometric/`.

11. `epiR`, created by Mark Stevenson with contributions from Telmo Nunes, Javier Sanchez, Ron Thornton, Jeno Reiczigel, Jim Robison-Cox and Paola Sebastiani, is a package for the analysis of epidemiological data. It contains functions for meta-analysis besides the typical usage for analysis of epidemiological data, such as directly and indirectly adjusting measures of disease frequency, quantifying measures of association on the basis of single or multiple strata of count data presented in a contingency table, and computing confidence intervals around incidence risk and incidence rate estimates. This package is available at `http://cran.r-project.org/web/packages/epiR/` or `http://epicentre.massey.ac.nz`.

12. `metamisc`, created by Thomas Debray, is a package for diagnostic and prognostic meta-analysis and is available at `http://cran.r-project.org/web/packages/metamisc/`. This package contains functions to estimate univariate, bivariate and multivariate models as well as allowing the aggregation of previously published prediction models with new data. A further description given in the package is, "The package provides tools for the meta-analysis of individual participant (IPD) and/or aggregate data (AD). Currently, it is possible to pool univariate summary (with `uvmeta`) and diagnostic accuracy (with `riley`) data. Whereas the former applies a univariate meta-analysis using DerSimonian and Laird's method (method-of-moment estimator), the latter implements a bivariate meta-analysis (Restricted Maximum Likelihood) using the alternative model for bivariate random-effects meta-analysis by Riley et al. (2008). For this the number of true positives (TP), false negatives (FN), true negatives (TN) and false positives (FP) for each study must be known."

13. `metaLik`, created by Annamaria Guolo and Cristiano Varin, is a package for likelihood inference in meta-analysis and meta-regression models and is available at `http://cran.r-project.org/web/packages/metaLik/`.

Finally,

14. `MADAM`, created by Karl Kugler, Laurin Mueller and Matthias Wieser, is a package that provides some basic methods for meta-analysis and is available at `http://cran.r-project.org/web/packages/MADAM/`. This package is aimed at implementing and improving meta-analysis methods used in biomedical research applications.

Bibliography

Adler, J. (2012). *R In a Nutshell, 2nd Edition.* Sebastopol, CA: O'Reilly Media, Inc.

Begg, C. B. and M. Mazumdar (1994). Operating characteristics of a rank correlation test for publication bias. *Biometrics 50*, 1088–1101.

Berkey, C. S., D. C. Hoaglin, A. Antezak-Bouckoms, F. Mosteller, and G. A. Colditz (1998). Meta-analysis of multiple outcomes by regression with random effects. *Statistics in Medicine 17*, 2537–2550.

Berkey, C. S., D. C. Hoaglin, F. Mosteller, and G. A. Colditz (1995). A random-effects regression model for meta-analysis. *Statistics in Medicine 14(4)*, 395–411.

Berman, N. G. and R. A. Parker (2002). Meta-analysis: Neither quick nor easy. *BMC Medical Research Methodology 2(10)*, 1–9.

Bhaumik, D. K., A. Amatya, S. T. Normand, J. Greenhouse, E. Kaizar, B. Neelon, and R. D. Gibbons (2012). Meta-analysis of rare binary adverse event data. *Journal of the American Statistical Association 107(498)*, 555–567.

Bohning, D., E. Dietz, P. Schlattmann, C. Viwatwonkasem, A. Biggeri, and J. Bock (2002). Some general points in estimating heterogeneity variance with the dersimonianŰlaird estimator. *Biostatistics 3*, 445–457.

Borenstein, M., L. V. Hedges, J. P. T. Higgins, and H. R. Rothstein (2009). *Introduction to Meta-Analysis.* West Sussex, United Kingdom: Wiley.

Cai, T., L. Parast, and L. Ryan (2010). Meta-analysis for rare events. *Statistics in Medicine 29(20)*, 2078–2089.

Calabrese, J. R., R. F. Huffman, R. L. White, S. Edwards, T. R. Thompson, and J. A. Ascher (2008). Lamotrigine in the acute treatment of bipolar depression: results of five double-blind, placebo-controlled clinical trials. *Bipolar Disorder 10*, 323–333.

Cannon, C. P., B. A. Steinberg, S. A. Murphy, J. L. Mega, and E. Braunwald (2006). Meta-analysis of cardiovascular outcomes trials comparing intensive versus moderate statin therapy. *Journal of the American College of Cardiology 48*, 438–445.

Chambers, J. M. (1998). *Programming with Data.* New York: Springer.

Chambers, J. M. (2008). *Software for Data Analysis: Programming with R.* New York: Springer.

Chen, D. G. and K. E. Peace (2010). *Clinical Trial Data Analysis Using R.* Boca Raton, FL: Chapman & Hall/CRC.

Chen, H., A. K. Manning, and J. Dupuis (2012). A method of moments estimator for random effect multivariate meta-analysis. *Biometrics*, (Epub May 2, 2012).

Cochran, W. G. (1952). The chi-squared test of goodness of fit. *Annals of Mathematical Statistics 23*, 315–345.

Cochran, W. G. (1954). The combination of estimates from different experiments. *Biometrics*, 101–129.

Cohen, J. (1988). *Statistical power analysis for the behavioral sciences (2nd ed.).* Hillsdale, NJ: Lawrence Erlbaum.

Colditz, G. A., T. F. Brewer, C. S. Berkey, M. E. Wilson, E. Burdick, H. V. Fineberg, and F. Mosteller (1994). Efficacy of bcg vaccine in the prevention of tuberculosis: Meta-analysis of the published literature. *Journal of the American Medical Association 271*, 698–702.

Cooper, H., L. V. Hedges, and J. C. Valentine (2009). *The Handbook of Research Synthesis and Meta-Analysis (2nd edition).* New York: Russell Sage Foundation.

Dahabreh, I. J. (2008). Meta-analysis of rare events: an update and sensitivity analysis of cardiovascular events in randomized trials of rosiglitazone. *Clinical Trials 5*, 116–120.

DerSimonian, R. and N. Laird (1986). Meta-analysis in clinical trials. *Controlled Clinical Trials 7*, 177–188.

Emerson, J. D. (1994). Combining estimates of the odds ratios: the state of the art. *Statistical Methods in Medical Research 3*, 157–178.

Everitt, B. and T. Hothorn (2006). *A Handbook of Statistical Analyses Using R.* Boca Raton, FL: Chapman & Hall/CRC.

Faraway, J. J. (2004). *Linear Models with R.* Boca Raton, FL: Chapman & Hall/CRC.

Faraway, J. J. (2006). *Extending Linear Models with R: Generalized Linear, Mixed Effects and Nonparametric Regression Models.* Boca Raton, FL: Chapman & Hall/CRC.

Field, A. P. (2003). The problems in using fixed-effects models of meta-analysis on real-world data. *Understanding Statistics 2*, 77–96.

Gardener, M. (2012). *Beginning R: The Statistical Programming Language.* Indianapolis, IN: John Wiley & Sons, Inc.

Gasparrini, A. Armstrong, B. and M. G. Kenward (2012). Multivariate meta-analysis for non-linear and other multi-parameter associations. *Statistics in Medicine Epub ahead of print*(doi: 10.1002/sim.5471).

Geddes, J. R., J. R. Calabrese, and G. M. Goodwin (2009). Lamotrigine for treatment of bipolar depression: independent meta-analysis and meta-regression of individual patient data from five randomized trials. *The British Journal of Psychiatry. 194*, 4–9.

Hardy, R. J. and S. G. Thompson (1998). Detecting and describing heterogeneity in meta-analysis. *Statistics in Medicine 17*, 841–856.

Hartung, J., G. Knapp, and B. K. Sinha (2008). *Statistical Meta-Analysis with Applications.* Hoboken, New Jersey: John Wiley & Sons, Inc.

Harwell, M. (1997). An empirical study of hedge's homogeneity test. *Psychological Methods 2*, 219–231.

Hedges, L. V. (1981). Distribution theory for glass's estimator of effect size and related estimators. *Journal of Educational Statistics 6*, 107–128.

Hedges, L. V. (1982). Estimating effect size from a series of independent experiments. *Psychological Bulletin 92*, 490–499.

Hedges, L. V. and I. Olkin (1985). *Statistical Methods for Meta-Analysis.* Orlando, FL: Academic Press, Inc.

Hedges, L. V. and J. L. Vevea (1998). Fixed- and random-effects models in meta-analysis. *Psychological Methods 3*, 486–504.

Higgins, J. P. T. and S. G. Thompson (2002). Quantifying heterogeneity in a meta-analysis. *Statistics in Medicine 21*, 1539–1558.

Higgins, J. P. T., S. G. Thompson, J. J. Deeks, and D. G. Altman (2003). Measuring inconsistency in meta-analyses. *British Medical Journal 327*, 557–560.

Huizenga, H. M., B. M. van Bers, J. Plat, W. P. van den Wildenberg, and M. W. van der Molen (2009). Task complexity enhances response inhibition deficits in childhood and adolescent attention-deficit /hyperactivity disorder: a meta-regression analysis. *Biological Psychiatry 65*, 39–45.

Hunter, J. E. and F. L. Schmidt (2004). *Methods of Meta-Analysis: Correcting Error and Bias in Research Findings. 2nd Edition.* Newbury Park, CA: Sage.

Ihaka, R. and R. Gentleman (1996). R: A language for data analysis and graphics. *Journal of Computational and Graphical Statistics 5(3)*, 299–314.

Kabacoff, R. I. (2011). *R In Action: Data Analysis and Graphics with R.* New York: Manning Publications Co.

Katcher, B. S. (2006). *MEDLINE: A Guide to Effective Searching in PubMed and Other Interfaces.* San Francisco, CA: Ashbury Press.

Lane, P. W. (2012). Meta-analysis of incidence of rare events. *Statistical Methods in Medical Research*, 2012 Jan 4 Epub.

Law, M. R., N. J. Wald, and S. G. Thompson (1994). By how much and how quickly does reduction in serum cholesterol concentration lower risk of ischaemic heart disease? *British Medical Journal 308*, 367–373.

Li, Y., L. Shi, and H. D. Roth (1994). The bias of the commonly-used estimate of variance in meta-analysis. *Communications in Statistics-Theory and Methods 23*, 1063–1085.

Lin, D. Y. and D. Zeng (2010). On the relative efficiency of the using summary statistics versus individual-level data in meta-analysis. *Biometrika 97(2)*, 321–332.

Lumley, T. (2009). rmeta: Meta-Analysis. R package version 2.16. URL http://CRAN.R-project.org/package=rmeta.

Lyman, G. H. and N. M. Kuderer (2005). The strengths and limitations of meta-analyses based on aggregate data. *BMC Medical Research Methodology 5*, 1–7.

Mantel, N. and W. Haenszel (1959). Statistical aspects of the analysis of data from retrospective studies of disease. *Journal of the National Cancer Institute 22(4)*, 719–748.

Marot, G., J.-L. Foulley, C.-D. Mayer, and F. Jaffrezic (2009). Moderated effect size and p-value combinations for microarray meta-analyses. *Bioinformatics 25(20)*, 2692–2699.

Mathew, T. and K. Nordstrom (1999). On the equivalence of meta-analysis using literature and using individual patient data. *Biometrics 55*, 1221–1223.

Morris, C. N. (1983). Parametric empirical bayes inference: Theory and applications (with discussion). *Journal of the American Statistical Association 78*, 47–65.

Murrell, P. (2005). *R Graphics.* Boca Raton, FL: Chapman & Hall/CRC.

Nissen, S. E. and K. Wolski (2007). Effect of rosiglitazone on the risk of myocardial infarction and death from cardiovascular causes. *The New England Journal of Medicine 356*, 2457–2471.

Normand, S. L. (1999). Meta-analysis: Formulating, evaluating, combining and reporting. *Statistics in Medicine 18*, 321–358.

Olkin, I. and A. Sampson (1998). Comparison of meta-analysis versus analysis of variance of individual patient data. *Biometrics 54*, 317–322.

Peace, K. E. (1991). Meta-analysis in ulcer disease. In *Swabb and Szabo (Eds.), Ulcer Disease: Investigation and basis for Therapy*, pp. 407–430. Marcel Dekker, Inc.

Peace, K. E. and D. G. Chen (2010). *Clinical Trial Methodology.* Boca Raton, FL: Chapman & Hall/CRC.

Petitti, D. B. (2000). *Meta-Analysis, Decision Analysis, and Cost-Effectiveness Analysis: Methods for Quantitative Synthesis in Medicine. 2nd Edition.* Oxford: Oxford University Press.

Pigott, T. D. (2012). *Advances in Meta-Analysis.* New York: Springer.

Riley, R. D., J. R. Thompson, and K. R. Abrams (2008). An alternative model for bivariate random-effects meta-analysis when the within-study correlations are unknown. *Biostatistics 9*, 172–186.

Rizzo, M. L. (2008). *Statistical Computing with R.* Boca Raton, FL: Chapman & Hall/CRC.

Roberts, C. and T. D. Stanley (2005). *Meta-Regression Analysis: Issues of Publication Bias in Economics.* Blackwell:Wiley.

Robins, J., N. Breslow, and S. Greenland (1986). Estimators of the mantel-haenszel variance consistent in both sparse data and large strata models. *Biometrics 42*, 311–323.

Rucker, G., G. Schwarzer, J. Carpenter, and I. Olkin (2009). Why add anything to nothing? the arcsine difference as a measure of treatment effect in meta-analysis with zero cells. *Statistics in Medicine 28(5)*, 721–738.

Sarkar, D. (2008). *Lattice: Multivariate Data Visualization with R.* New York: Springer.

Schulze, R. (2004). *Meta-analysis: a comparison of approaches.* Gottingen, Germany:Hogrefe & Huber.

Schwarzer, G. (2010). meta: Meta-Analysis with R. R package version 1.6-0, URL http://CRAN.R-project.org/package=meta.

Shuster, J. J., L. S. Jones, and D. A. Salmon (2007). Fixed vs random effects meta-analysis in rare event studies: the rosiglitazone link with myocardial infarction and cardiac death. *Statistics in Medicine 26(24)*, 4375–4385.

Shuster, J. J. and D. A. Schatz (2008). The rosigliazone meta-analysis: Lessons for the future. *Diabetes Care 31(3), March 2008*, 10.

Sidik, K. and J. N. Jonkman (2005a). A note on variance estimation in random effects meta-regression. *Journal of Biopharmaceutical Statistics 15*, 823–838.

Sidik, K. and J. N. Jonkman (2005b). Simple heterogeneity variance estimation for meta-analysis. *Journal of the Royal Statistical Society, Series C, 54*, 367–384.

Simmonds, M. C. and J. P. T. Higgins (2007). Covariate heterogeneity in meta-analysis: Criteria for deciding between meta-regression and individual patient data. *Statistics in Medicine 26*, 2982–2999.

Simmonds, M. C., J. P. T. Higgins, L. A. Stewartb, J. F. Tierneyb, M. J. Clarke, and S. G. Thompson (2005). Meta-analysis of individual patient data from randomized trials: a review of methods used in practice. *Clinical Trials 2*, 209–217.

Singh, K., M. Xie, and W. E. Strawderman (2005). Combining information from independent sources through confidence distribution. *Annals of Statistics 33*, 159–183.

Sutton, A. J., N. J. Cooper, P. C. Lambert, D. R. Jones, K. R. Abrams, and M. J. Sweeting (2002). Meta-analysis of rare and adverse event data. *Expert Review of Pharmacoeconomics and Outcomes Research 2(4)*, 367–379.

Sutton, A. J. and J. P. T. Higgins (2008). Recent developments in meta-analysis. *Statistics in Medicine 27*, 625–650.

Sweeting, M. J., A. J. Sutton, and P. C. Lambert (2004). What to add to nothing? use and avoidance of continuity corrections in meta-analysis of sparse data. *Statistics in Medicine 23*, 1351–1375.

Thompson, S. G. and J. P. T. Higgins (2002). How should meta-regression analyses be undertaken and interpreted? *Statistics in Medicine 21(11)*, 1559–1573.

Thompson, S. G. and S. Sharp (1999). Explaining heterogeneity in meta-analysis: a comparison of methods. *Statistics in Medicine 18*, 2693–2708.

Tian, L., T. Cai, M. Pfeffer, N. Piankov, P. Cremieux, and L. Wei (2009). Exact and efficient inference procedure for meta-analysis and its application to the analysis of independent 2 by 2 tables with all available data but without artificial continuity correction. *Biostatistics 10(2)*, 275–281.

van Houwelingen, H. C., L. R. Arends, and T. Stijnen (2002). Tutorial in biostatistics: Advanced methods in meta-analysis: Multivariate approach and meta-regression. *Statistics in Medicine 21*, 589–624.

Viechtbauer, W. (2005). Bias and efficiency of meta-analytic variance estimators in the random-effects model. *Journal of Educational and Behavioral Statistics 30*, 261–293.

Viechtbauer, W. (2010). Conducting meta-analyses in R with the *metafor* package. *Journal of Statistical Software 36(1)*, 1–48.

Wang, J., C. Zhao, Z. C., X. Fan, Y. Lin, and Q. Jiang (2011). Tubeless vs standard percutaneous nephrolithotomy: a meta-analysis. *British Journal of Urology International 109*, 918–924.

West, S., V. King, T. S. Carey, K. N. Lohr, N. McKoy, S. F. Sutton, and L. Lux (2002). Systems to Rate the Strength of Scientific Evidence. Evidence Report/Technology Assessment No. 47 (Prepared by the Research Triangle Institute-University of North Carolina Evidence-based Practice Center under Contract No. 290-97-0011). *In AHRQ Publication No. 02-E016. Rockville, MD: Agency for Healthcare Research and Quality*, 64–88.

Whitehead, A. (2003). *Meta-Analysis of Controlled Clinical Trials.* New York, NY:John Wiley & Sons, Inc.

Whitehead, A., A. J. Bailey, and D. Elbourne (1999). Combining summaries of binary outcomes with those of continuous outcomes in a meta-analysis. *Journal of Biopharmaceutical Statistics 9*(1), 1–16.

Xie, M. and K. Singh (2013). Confidence distribution, the frequentist distribution estimator of a parameter – a review. *International Statistical Review.*, In Press.

Xie, M., K. Singh, and W. E. Strawderman (2011). Confidence distributions and a unifying framework for meta-analysis. *Journal of the American Statistical Association 106*, 320–333.

Yusuf, S., R. Peto, J. Lewis, R. Collins, and P. Sleight (1985). Beta blockade during and after myocardial infarction: an overview of the randomized trials. *Progress in Cardiovascular Diseases 27*, 335–371.

Index